How to be a SuperAger

You Can Make the Rest of Your Life the Best of Your Life

John Owen

Important Notice and Disclaimer

AGING

Is the Failing
Ability of the Body
to Defend, Maintain,
and Repair Itself.

GREY DOG BOOKS

Published by Grey Dog Books, Tulsa, OK

CONTENTS

Cognitive abilities, particularly memory, normally decline with age. However, some individuals, often designated as SuperAgers, can reach late life with the memory function of individuals 30 years younger.

Garo-Pascual, Gase, et al, The Lancet, 2023

A SuperAger is someone age 80 or older who exhibits cognitive function that is comparable to an average person who is middle aged.

Lee A. Lindquist, Northwestern University
Feinberg School of Medicine website

Introduction

To learn the secrets of a SuperAger, you need to learn about your body from the inside out. Every minute of your life, your heart contracts around 75 times, pumping about five liters of blood through blood vessels ranging in thickness from the size of a cigar to less than the width of a single hair. Each minute, 25 trillion blood cells will pass through your arteries, veins, and capillaries, a distance of 60,000 miles, supplying oxygen and nutrients to all parts of your body. Also, during this minute, about 120 million of your red blood cells will die. Fortunately, your body will make 120 million new ones to replace them.

These are staggering numbers. Are these miracles? Your 60,000 miles of blood vessels is long enough to wrap around the earth twice, with 10,000 miles left over. The lining of your intestines is completely replaced every three to five days, while, at the same time, your body takes a cheeseburger, a Dr. Pepper, and a pack of Twinkies and turns them into testosterone, blood, insulin, thyroid, skin, hair, sperm, intestinal lining, and more. In 90 to 120 days your body produces more than 37 trillion new cells– enough to make a whole new you. Now *that's* a miracle!

In this book you'll learn a lot of surprising facts about your body and, even better, you'll learn how you can make a real difference in your health and life expectancy. Your body chemistry is in total control of your future. Your body's chemistry is very complex, containing a staggering number of chemicals that interact with each other. There are four things that affect your body chemistry: what you eat, what you do, what you inherited from your parents (genes), and the environment you live in. If you're an average person who doesn't always eat right or exercise enough. If you're a person who wants to get better but isn't ready to jump into the latest fitness-diet fad, a person who wants some basic information about how your body works and how you can make some progress in the right direction without looking stupid, you're in the right place. Keep reading!

Basically, you're a walking pharmaceutical factory. The thousands of chemicals produced in your body, by your body, constantly interact with each other. Sometimes that's healthy, sometimes decidedly not. All of them are necessary: inflammation is your body's defense against infection, but if it is too strong or hangs around too long it can hurt your body. That's why your body has anti-inflammatory substances. The trick to keeping it all in good working order is to have everything in balance with both inflammatory and anti-inflammatory chemicals, coagulant and anticoagulant chemicals, oxidant and antioxidant chemicals, vasodilators (they make blood vessels larger) and vasoconstrictors (they make blood vessels smaller), and so on. Medical people have a fancy word for this state of balance— homeostasis.

If you can say
Romeo Stacy, then you can say **homeostasis**

Homeostasis is a very important word. It's a self-regulating process by which the body tries to maintain balance, stability and survival while adjusting to conditions that your body encounters. If homeostasis is successful, life continues, but if it's unsuccessful, it can result in deterioration or death. *The goal of all medicine is to restore your body to this condition —**homeostasis!***

This book is designed to help you understand how your body works and how you can take control. You will learn some more big words like homeostasis, along with how to say them and what they mean for your body and your health. You will learn how—

Walking can increase the cells (neurons) in your brain.

Walking can decrease the odds of getting Alzheimer's

Walking can decrease the odds of getting Parkinson's Disease.

Walking can decrease the possibility of falls (33 million Americans fall annually.)

Walking can delay or prevent type 2 diabetes.

Walking can decrease inflammation.

Walking can increase mitochondria.

Walking can help heal wounds.

Walking can improve your mood and reduce depression.

Walking can improve your cardiovascular health.

Walking can lower your blood pressure.

Walking can help you lose weight.

Walking can prevent weakness and muscle wasting.

Walking can help you feel better.

Walking can improve your lungs and breathing capacity.

Walking can give you more energy.

Walking can move you toward **homeostasis** (hey, you know that word!)

Walking can improve and extend your life.

Walking can flip the switch, changing your body chemistry from unhealthy to healthy, feeling bad to feeling good, from shorter life to longer life. **Just walking!**

The deep dive

You will learn what myokines, hemodynamics, epigenetics, and mechanotransduction are (more big words we will explain), then you'll learn how to use them to change your blood chemistry. All the information will be in everyday English with only a few big words to learn. (Some big words, however, are just too much to explain and I will use initials with a reference so you can explore the meaning if you wish.) There are simple illustrations to help you grasp the meanings, as well as references to source documents for the academic readers. Information is drawn primarily from the National Institute of Health's database of peer-reviewed articles called PubMed, as well as major university medical schools and national news sources. If websites are referenced, you will be given the web addresses.

Along the way, you will discover the exact things you need to do to switch your body chemistry from bad to good. It does require some effort but not so much that an out-of-shape grandfather can't do it. You may even find, as this out-of-shape grandfather did, that you actually enjoy it.

As Dr, Seuss wisely said,

"You have brains in your head. You have feet in your shoes.
You can steer yourself any direction you choose.
You're on your own. And you know what you know.
And YOU are the one who'll decide where to go..."

So, let's get going!

1

It all begins with My Toe Sis and ends with Zombies

Identical twins we'll call Sarah and Susan posed a real mystery to researchers in England a few years ago. When exhaustive biometric measurements were taken, the sisters were discovered to be exactly the same in all respects. During their years in the study, however, Susan's brain became smaller and unhealthy compared to Sarah's. Susan's smaller brain led, unsurprisingly, to reduced cognition and function whereas Sarah's larger brain continued to function normally. Susan also suffered from weakness.

In addition to their examination of physiological and cardiovascular risk factors such as cholesterol and blood pressure, researchers examined small details of the twins' lives. The twins grew up in the same house, had similar diets, and attended the same schools. Both married at about the same age and had remarkably similar husbands and families. Their careers were also similar. Neither was subject to more stress in their life, and neither was exposed to unique environmental hazards.

When they went back to reexamine their data in greater detail, the researchers found only one small difference — Sarah had better leg muscles. There, at last, they found their answer: Sarah walked a lot and Susan was sedentary! That small detail was the deciding factor in their vastly different mental conditions as they aged.

The researchers conducting the study know a lot about twins. They are a part of the Twin Project conducted by The Department of Twin Research and Genetic Epidemiology at King's College, London. The project has, since 1992, studied more than 14,000 twins. Their mission, as stated on their website, is to "investigate the genetic and environmental basis of complex diseases and conditions to understand how genetic variation relates to human health". They have amassed a remarkable amount of genetic data.

How, you might ask, does leg strength relate to cognitive health as people age? According to Claire Steves, PhD, the geriatrician who heads the Twin Research & Genetic Epidemiology department, brain imaging was done at the beginning of the study. Years later, when imaging was done again, Sarah, the twin with the stronger legs had more gray matter and more white matter with less empty space in the skull. "Looking at the X-rays, you don't need to be a neuroscientist to see that the empty spaces are much smaller in the stronger twin than in the weaker twin," Dr. Steves said. And most people will probably agree that you don't have to be a neuroscientist to know that having empty spaces in your brain is a bad thing!

You don't have to be a neuroscientist to know that empty spaces in your brain are bad for you!

Why was Sarah's brain larger? Because, when you walk, your legs pump blood to your brain delivering more oxygen and nutrients to feed your brain, helping it to function and thrive. The legs are sometimes called "the muscle pump," or "the second heart," because they have a system of muscles, veins, and one-way valves in the calf and foot that work together to push blood back up to the heart and lungs. The vein valves open and close with each muscle contraction to prevent the backflow of blood.

We all lose muscle mass and strength beginning around the age of 30 and progressing at approximately three to eight percent per decade. The rate of decline is even higher after the age of 60. This is why we all need exercise: to slow or prevent this decline. In the case of the twins, Sarah's walking apparently protected her from at least some of these problems since she didn't exhibit any symptoms of frailty and weakness. Susan's lack of walking, on the other hand, resulted in muscle wasting (sarcopenia) which contributes to frailty and falls. The U.S. Centers for Disease Control and Prevention (CDC) reports that more than 25 percent of all Americans over the age of 65 will fall each year.

By her practice of walking, Sarah was not only supplying more blood, oxygen, and nutrients to the brain, but the moving blood caused profound changes in her body chemistry through a magical process called mechanotransduction. Don't let that word scare you. If you can say mechanic transmission, it's almost the same thing. Let's just call it transduction.

When blood is flowing through your arteries, the moving blood cells create friction with the lining of that vessel, called the endothelium. The cells forming the endothelium respond to this friction by producing chemicals. It's kind of like rubbing something to create static electricity—which is another kind of transduction.

What kinds of chemicals? Many helpful substances such as antioxidants, anti-inflammatories, and anti-coagulants. Walking also causes the muscles to produce several myokines, which are small messenger proteins, that can help reduce the chemicals (tau and amyloid beta) that cause Alzheimer's Disease and Parkinson's Disease. Marc Milstein, PhD, author of *The Age Proof Brain*, says, "Simply walking is really important for your brain health and people who walk 30 minutes a day can lower their risk of dementia by about 60 percent."

According to *Walking for Health*, published by Harvard Medical School, you can lower your blood pressure, fight heart disease, reduce the risk for diabetes, relieve depression, improve memory, and add healthy years to your life, just by walking! Harvard advertises the booklet as "The simple cure for the biggest health problems in America."

Does this mean that you can delay or even escape cognitive decline just by walking? Well yes, it probably does. It depends on your current health and age, any other medical conditions you may have and how faithfully you adhere to the requirements of your walking routine. There are some requirements, of course. You should walk at least 150 minutes a week at a brisk pace of about 100 steps per minute. That's about the tempo of *Stayin' Alive* by the BeeGees, or *Another One Bites the Dust*, by Queen, or, as The American Heart Association recently pointed out, *The Man* by Taylor Swift. You can walk 30 minutes a day for five days or 15 ten-minute sessions scattered throughout the week.

"Exercise is the most important thing you can do to maintain your cognitive health."

Dr. Sharon Inouye, Director
Harvard University Medical School / Aging Brain Center

Isn't it amazing what a little friction in your blood vessels can do? To help you understand that better, let's take a look at the processes in your body that make this possible.

In the Beginning . . .

A new life begins when a sperm meets an egg and penetrates it, creating a single cell called a zygote. Researchers report a visible spark when this happens! Around 30 hours later, the cell divides into two cells, then, 15 hours later, the two divide into four. This process keeps repeating for the next nine months or so, until there are about 37 trillion cells, comprising a complete human. This process of cell division is called mitosis (my TOE sis).

Mitosis does not end once a person is complete, because almost all the cells in your body are constantly dying and being replaced, mostly through mitosis. We have already mentioned that red blood cells last around 100 days. White blood cells, on the other hand, live only a few days. Your skin cells live for a month or so. Eventually, however, some cells just get tired of mitosis and stop dividing. This can create problems. There is a process called apoptosis (apo-TOE-sis [the second p is silent]) that leads to the removal and recycling or disposal of the dying cell. In simple terms, it's taking out the trash. The word apoptosis was introduced in 1972, by John Kerr, and colleagues, who coined the term from the Greek apo plus ptosis, meaning falling off, in the same way that fruit falls from a tree when it becomes ripe. Apoptosis happens normally during development and aging and as a mechanism to maintain cell populations in tissues.

Toward the end of your life, some cells quit dividing and then instead of reporting to the recycling/disposal center for apotosis, they hang around as "zombie" cells. These non-working cells become toxic, literally, by emitting toxins that damage other cells. Zombie cells are called senescent, (sen-ESS-unt) and, eventually, can signal the approaching end of your life. Your dying cells are not being replaced

The concept of senescence was discovered in the 1960's when two researchers (Hayflick and Moorhead) observed that after a number of divisions, certain cells entered an "irreversible state of growth arrest" (no mitosis). Since then, many research teams have become interested in determining the hallmarks of cell senescence, the factors that induce it, the effect of senescence on other cells and the body as a whole. While there are many research projects to define new causes of senescence, we know that senescence can be induced by damage to DNA, shortening of telomeres (the protective caps at the end of DNA molecules), mitochondrial damage, and something called epigenetic factors, which refers to changes that affect the way DNA is packaged and genes are expressed.

Many scientists believe that aging is a disease that can be cured, or at least postponed for a significant time. To that end, many researchers are working toward a drug that will be senolytic, which means something that will stop senescence.

Among the best known of these researchers is Aubrey de Grey, a PhD gerontologist from Cambridge University (who looks like a backup guitarist for ZZ Top), and the chairman of the aptly named Methuselah Foundation. He wrote a book titled, *Ending Aging, the rejuvenation breakthroughs that could reverse human aging in our lifetimes.* On the cover is a picture of an hourglass, but with the sand flowing up! He coined the term SENS, an acronym for Strategies for Engineered Negligible Senescence.

While the entire discussion about anti-aging and the extraordinary scientific advancements that are developing is beyond the scope of this book, I felt compelled to include some of it because I ran across a peer-reviewed article with a title that that spoke to me: "Is exercise a senolytic medicine? A systematic review." Here's the quote that caught my eye:

"Exercise is a potent anti-aging and anti-chronic disease medicine, which has shown the capacity to lower the markers of cellular senescence over the past decade... Here, we have conducted a systematic review of the published literature, studying the senolytic effects of exercise or physical activity

on senescent cells under various states in humans. *Exercise can reduce senescent cells in healthy humans."*
(Chen et al, 2020)

What? You mean that we can put the brakes on senescence just by walking? Holy cow! Does Aubrey know about this? It's not the full answer of course, but it's a step in the right direction. Several steps, actually. *Ending Aging* explains the major classes of life-long accumulating damage that bring about the life-ending effects of aging, and in later sections of this book, we'll show how you can reduce some of them by walking. De Grey's earlier book, *The Mitochondrial Free Radical Theory of Aging* basically makes the argument that free radicals (another name for oxidants) produced by mitochondria cause mitochondrial dysfunction, the bad effects of aging and, ultimately, death.

If you can say **My Toe Laundry On**, then change one
letter to say **My Toe Kaundry On**,
then you can say **Mitochondrion**. In fact, you just did!

Just as trains, planes, and automobiles need fuel to run, your body runs on a fuel called ATP (adenosine triphosphate). How much of this fuel do you burn every day? It varies with your size and activity, of course, but generally, you produce and burn your bodyweight in ATP every 24 hours. You may be thinking, "How can this be? I don't even eat 150 pounds of food a day!" And you would be partly right. The ATP produced in your body is derived from your food, but the process is able to recycle the basic chemicals derived from your food several times, extracting energy each time. It's pure magic from an organelle (small organ) called the mitochondrion.

Mitochondria [plural] power your life. They are your inner power plant. You have trillions of these incredibly small organelles that perform complex atomic-level mechanical and electro-chemical procedures that are almost beyond understanding. They are the mini-factories producing all your ATP. Mitochondria are found in most cells in your body. How many in each cell? It varies. You may find anywhere from a handful, to more than 2000 of them in each cell. Since you have 37 trillion cells in your body, we're talking about a mind-boggling number of them (a gazillion?). I would strongly suggest that you watch some of the many videos on YouTube that use some excellent animation techniques to explain how mitochondria work.

Here are a few:

"Mitochondria Aren't Just the Powerhouse of the Cell" https://youtu.be/1xwaG-GBHIU

"ATP Synthase in Action" https://youtu.be/A2my52zQA6k

"Electron Transport Chain" https://youtu.be/rdF3mnyS1p0

"The Molecular Basis of Life" https://youtu.be/fpHaxzroYxg

Spoiler alert: after watching two, or three, or twenty videos, don't be surprised to find that you still don't understand mitochondria. But at least you'll have a clearer appreciation for these elegantly complex organelles that work tirelessly every second to keep you alive.

Once, on a day with sub-freezing weather, rain, sleet, and snow, I decided to do my walking indoors and headed to a local mall. I put on earphones and prepared to walk by selecting a program on YouTube. (We'll talk more about the many things you can do while walking). The program I selected was a talk given at the University of Texas in Galveston, by Bret Goodpaster, an aging expert who has published more than 200 peer-reviewed articles. The talk was, *"Mitochondrial Energetics and Insulin Resistance in Aging."* (Yes, I know that a "normal" person doesn't walk around a mall listening to such stuff, but I really don't identify as "normal").

About 40 minutes into his talk, he said something that made me stop, and say out loud, "Wait, what?" He said that researchers had taken a group of older adults and enrolled them in a program where they walked briskly for 30 to 40 minutes, three times a week, for 12 weeks. Afterward, they measured several aspects of their mitochondrial performance and found that their mitochondria increased by more than 50%." That's astounding! It's called mitochondrial biogenesis.

When I got home, I watched the program (walking, I could only listen to it) and when he made that remark, I saw that he was displaying a slide with a bar chart and the referenced research

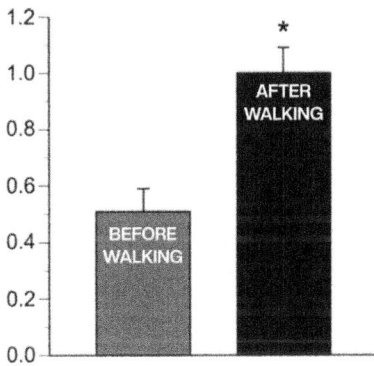

article. I found the article on the National Institute of Health's database of scientific articles called PubMed.gov (by Menshikova, et al 2006, *Journal of Gerontology*). I printed it, read it, and came away convinced that this was the real deal. Here's the mitochondria chart from the article.

At this time, you know that we all have about a gazillion mitochondria, and these older adults had just added half a gazillion shiny, brand new, functional mitochondria by walking for 12 weeks? Doesn't it seem reasonable to believe that a person with that many new, healthy mitochondria might have better prospects for longevity? Walking is starting to look like serious medicine, right? What if they didn't stop, but just kept on walking?

That brings us to 95-year-old Olga Kotelko, whose story I found in the New York Times. She was considered one of the world's greatest athletes, who held 30 world records and 750 gold medals in track and field. At a championship event in Finland, Olga threw a javelin more than 20 feet farther than her nearest age-group rival. At the World Masters Games in Sydney, her time in the 100 meters was faster than that of some finalists in the 80- to-84-year category, two brackets down.

Olga came to athletics late in life. She taught in a one-room schoolhouse, then moved to British Columbia with her two daughters and brought them up while earning her bachelor's degree at night. She picked up softball after retiring from teaching, and when she was 77, a teammate suggested she might enjoy track and field.

She found a coach who taught her the basics. Then she found a trainer — a strict Hungarian woman who pushed her hard. Until her death at 95 she still did some hard training including three sets of 10 push-ups and three sets of 25 sit-ups daily.

Physical activity such as walking can help you think, learn, problem-solve, improve memory, and reduce anxiety or depression. It can also reduce your risk of cognitive decline, including dementia.

CDC Website

Tanja Taivassalo, PhD, is a physiologist at McGill University in Toronto, whose area of expertise is mitochondrial research; she examines what happens to the body when mitochondria are faulty. She has studied Olga extensively. When Olga's first muscle samples came back from the lab, the results were compelling. In a muscle sample of a person over the age of 65, even more so at 95, you would normally see some mitochondrial defects. But in

400 of Olga's muscle fibers examined, Taivassalo said, "we didn't see a single fiber that had any evidence" of mitochondrial decay. "It's remarkable," she added.

Apparently, Olga was doing something to hold off senescence and retain healthy mitochondrial function. If Aubrey de Grey and others are correct, Olga should have had many senescent cells. In chapter three, we'll do a mini lesson on the cardiovascular system plus an introduction to what I call "your inner pharmaceutical factory" which may be the thing that enabled Olga to beat the odds and can help you do the same.

This book is divided into chapters that are heavy on information about science and physiology and others that are about some practical (and impractical) aspects of walking. This is done in a shameless attempt to keep you reading. Shielding you from experiencing a brain overload or, on the other hand, boredom.

2

Pumping Blood, Mechanic, Transmission. . . Magic!

When your heart contracts, it pumps blood through your cardiovascular circulation system. Blood flows out of the heart through your arteries. It returns via your veins. In between are the capillaries (Cappy Larry's). By the time your blood gets to your capillaries it has lost the pumping effects from your heart, meaning that it is not pulsing, but flowing continuously, and very weakly. In fact, in much of the body, it does not have enough force to return to your heart. The way that blood returns is through something called the "muscle pump." In the veins of your feet and legs, there are small one-way valves that let the blood flow toward the heart while preventing it from flowing backward. As your muscles contract, they squeeze the veins and move the blood along in a manner similar to the way you squeeze toothpaste from a tube. This process effectively "pumps" blood back to the heart.

Your heart pumps around five liters of blood (1-1/3 gallons) per minute and since your body contains about five liters of blood, your blood circulates about once a minute. As you increase your activities through walking or other exercise the flow is accelerated. If you are sedentary, on the other hand, the flow slows.

a human hair
about 70 microns

a human capillary
about 4 to 9 microns

red blood cell
7.5 to 8.7 microns

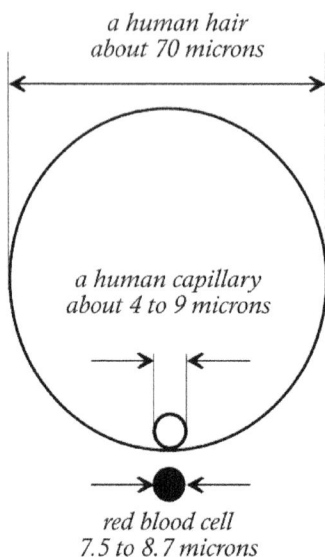

The purpose of blood circulation is to deliver oxygen and nutrients (and any medications you may be using) to your cells. Your arteries and arterioles have walls with three layers of tissue. But when we get to the capillaries, they have a single layer which has microscopic openings in it allowing small molecules such as oxygen and vitamins, to pass into the cellular spaces, and waste products to pass into the capillaries for disposal. How small are capillaries? Smaller than many of the red blood cells that must pass through them. Smaller than you would ever guess. About 70 of them would fit within a single human hair. Many of the red blood cells have to fold and bend in order to pass through. Some diseases, such as diabetes, cause the red blood cells to be stiff, or less flexible, ("reduced erythrocyte deformability" in doctor talk) which makes some diseases worse through reduced circulation, increased coagulation and a greater risk of blood clots.

The *movement* of your blood exerts an incredible influence on your body chemistry. As the blood flows along, it creates friction between the blood cells and the endothelium which triggers a magical process we have mentioned before, called **mechanotransduction**.

If you can say **mechanic transmission,**
then you can say
mechano transduction, right?

This is Important.
Mechanotransduction Is a Big Deal!

I'm afraid, however, that mechanotransduction may be a little awkward to read, so I will just call it transduction in the rest of the book. Transduction causes the endothelial cells to release chemicals. It's sort of like rubbing something to create static electricity, except in this case, you're creating chemicals. The *friction* from the blood as it passes the vessel wall, is called ***shear stress****,* and it causes the cells lining your blood vessels to produce chemicals. Hundreds of them! This little-known process, your

Blood vessel showing mechanotransduction

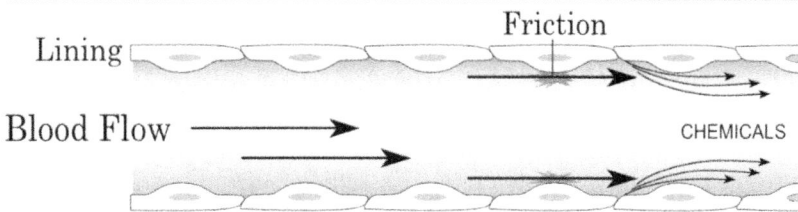

Friction

Lining

Blood Flow ⟶

CHEMICALS

chemical-production facility, is the key to what I call your "inner pharmaceutical factory." But here's the important part: *high*

(normal) blood flow and shear stress, which comes from physical activities, creates good, healthy chemicals whereas *low blood flow and shear stress,* the result of sedentary living, creates bad, unhealthy chemicals. It's almost like flipping a switch. If you're active (by walking, for example) you stay healthier. If you're a couch potato, your body chemistry will become your enemy and you are likely to meet your maker earlier than those walking people.

If you can say **Elmo Helium**
you can say **endothelium**

The lining of your blood vessels is called the endothelium and is made up of endothelial cells. Working independently, Louis Ignarro, Robert Furchgott, and Ferid Murad discovered an unknown substance produced by endothelial cells that relaxes blood vessels. Initially, it was called "endothelium-derived relaxing factor" (EDRF) then in 1978, Ignarro discovered that the mysterious EDRF was a gas named **nitric oxide**. Ignarro, Furchgott and Murad received a Nobel Prize for discovering "nitric oxide as a signaling molecule in the cardiovascular system".

Ignarro first announced his results at a meeting of his doctor-scientist peers, and, to his surprise, they laughed! The problem with them believing him was not only that nitric oxide is a gas, but it disappears in about a second. How, they asked, could this rapidly disappearing gas affect the blood vessels? For several years, some of his peers argued in published papers that he was wrong, but today, it is accepted as a fact. Nitric Oxide has turned out to be an extremely important molecule in the operation of our bodies. In 1992, it was named "Molecule of the Year" by *Science Magazine*.

Nitric oxide is so important that the *lack* of it is the basic definition of endothelial dysfunction. When nitric oxide is made, it permeates adjacent muscle tissues in less than a second, causing arteries to relax and expand, thereby increasing blood flow and reducing blood pressure. Nitric oxide also signals immune cells to kill harmful bacteria and cancer cells and helps brain cells to communicate with each other. It reduces the inflammation of arthritis, protects bones from osteoporosis, helps heal chronic wounds, is essential for both male and female sexual functions, and much more.

Researchers in 1998 (Traub and Berk) used a drug to increase nitric oxide which elevated it as much as 600 percent. On the other hand, when they boosted blood flow and shear stress, nitric oxide increased as much as 3,000 percent! They clearly demonstrated that *the strongest stimulus for creation of nitric oxide is blood flow, shear stress and transduction* — which you can create in your body by *walking.*

Whenever you do a moderate-intensity activity, whether it's walking, jogging, dancing, bicycling, gardening, shopping — anything that elevates your blood flow — your body responds to the increased blood flow by remodeling your blood vessels outward to accommodate the new, higher levels of blood flow. Let me say that again — when you engage in physical activity, your body makes your blood vessels larger to accommodate the additional blood flow. This doesn't take place overnight, but continued physical activity over time will cause this to happen, and your new vascular system will deliver more blood, oxygen, and nutrients to your tissues. *Walking remodels your vascular system* making it healthier so it can better support your muscles, heart, lung and, well, everything in your body, thus helping you to become healthier. It's helping you move toward **homeostasis**.

A couple of other things are happening at the same time to further improve blood circulation.

First, there is a process called **arteriogenesis**, which means "growth of new arteries" that can be stimulated by increases in blood flow and shear stress. There are millions of little "connector tubes" called **anastomoses** (say Canasta Moses without the C) normally in the body serving as backup routes for blood flow if a blood vessel is blocked or otherwise compromised. These little stand-by blood vessels, flat and empty, just waiting till you need them, can be activated (enlarged up to 2,000 percent) by increased blood flow and shear stress as well as nitric oxide and VEGF, all of which are increased by walking. The newly developed blood vessels are called "collateral circulation." They will not carry as much blood as your original blood vessels, but they are usually good enough to feed your tissues.

The second thing that happens is called **angiogenesis**, which means "growth of new capillaries." The triggering effect for this is a signal from the muscle cells that they need oxygen. They might need oxygen because they are ischemic (have too little blood supply) or because the muscles are contracting which creates a demand for more oxygen and nutrients (mainly glucose, which is sugar). Once the body receives this message, it responds by sending more blood to the tissue cells.

The effects of blood flow on your endothelium is critical for your health through an array of physiological functions, and we will discuss it more in subsequent chapters.

Shifting goals for exercise as we age

Now that you understand the importance of blood flow, transduction and the work of your inner pharmaceutical factory, you need to think about the exercises most likely to promote circulation and all its many benefits. Since your muscle pump with all its one-way valves can be found in your lower legs, do you think that would be the best place to focus your exercise? Of course it would. Having big biceps, flat or six-pack abs, or even a thinner, more shapely figure might all be reasonable goals for younger people, but today you need to ask your self this question: will any of those things help you live a longer and healthier life? Well, maybe a little, but not much.

If you want to be healthier and extend your life through blood flow and the hundreds of chemical changes that come with that, you need to walk, run, dance, jump rope, hike, play tennis, pickleball or *whatever pumps blood!* Bench presses, curls, squats, planking are not the best types of exercises for promoting cardiovascular circulation. Walking is probably the best choice for blood flow because almost everyone can do it, it can be included in your daily routine, you don't need special clothing or equipment, it specifically targets the muscle pump, and it's free.

Here is an example, one of many, that shows two benefits of walking:

Walking can increase the size of your brain and improve your memory

The hippocampus — the part of your brain that deals with memory and learning — shrinks in late life, leading to impaired memory and increased risk for dementia. Your hippocampus shrinks one to two percent annually, and this loss of brain volume increases the risk for cognitive impairment.

— *From the Proceedings of the National Academy of Sciences*

Yes, we all experience brain shrinkage as we age, but research shows that we can reverse it with just a little effort. A group of researchers from the University of Pittsburgh, University of Illinois, Ohio State University, and Rice University, in a randomized, controlled trial of 120 *older adults*, found that brisk walking (100 steps per minute, 150 minutes a week), could make a real difference in the way our brains age.

Over time, you can change your future brain size

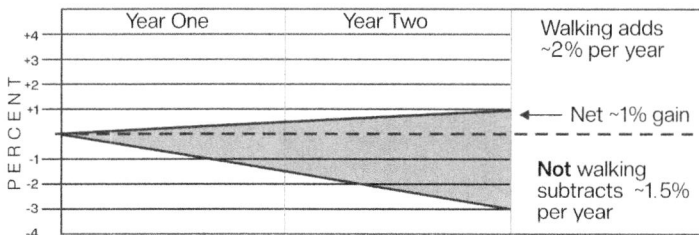

Our results demonstrate that the size of the hippocampus is modifiable in late adulthood and that moderate-intensity aerobic exercise is effective at reversing volume loss.

In the study, they found that one year of aerobic exercise (specifically walking but not stretching) increased hippocampus size by about two percent, offsetting the deterioration associated with aging. Because the hippocampus shrinks at a rate of one to two percent annually, a two percent increase in hippocampus volume is equivalent to adding one to two years of volume to the hippocampus. Or, in other words, it's like subtracting age from your brain!

"In sum, we found that the hippocampus remains plastic — has the ability to change, grow and learn — in late life and one year of moderate aerobic exercise (walking) was sufficient for enhancing volume. Increased hippocampus volume translates to improved memory function and higher serum levels of a chemical called Brain-Derived Neuroptophic Factor (BDNF), which protects brain cells and helps to grow new ones. We also demonstrated that higher fitness levels are protective against hippocampus shrinkage."

Walking is really important for your brain health and it doesn't cost a thing.

Marc Milstein, The Age Proof Brain

The study showed that the group which was randomized to stretching exercises experienced about a 1.5 percent decline in hippocampus size in one year, while those in the walking group experienced about a 2 percent increase in size per year, for a net increase of a half percent per year. The cumulative effect clearly establishes a **trajectory** where, in the future, the *walking you* could have a larger and better functioning brain than the *sedentary you*. In twenty years your brain could be 30% smaller or 10% larger. The only difference is walking — and you can choose which trajectory you want. I can't think of any other exercise that offers such a clear benefit in return for such a small investment of your time and energy.

All this scientific study validates the real-life example of the twin sisters in chapter one. The old saying—*use it or lose it*—is certainly true of your brain.

Their concluding statement, below, should give us all a reason to get out there and start walking!

These results clearly indicate that aerobic exercise is neuroprotective and that starting an exercise regimen later in life is not futile for either enhancing cognition or augmenting brain volume.

Exercise Goals for the SuperAger

1. To increase blood flow that delivers oxygen and nutrients to cells

2. To create endothelial shear stress/friction leading to transduction

3. To increase muscle contractions leading to the release of myokines

In succeeding chapters we will explain these exercise goals

3

Walking is the Perfect Exercise

If you search for the benefits of exercise, you will find a long list of diseases and physical conditions that are improved or reversed by walking. Unfortunately, many of these stories fail to explain exactly how that process works. In chapter one, the twins story explained how transduction and myokines were produced in response to walking, (muscle contractions) and the effect that had on their brains. But the story of how this process works is much larger than that.

For instance, two of my favorite molecules are KLF2 and Nrf2 (they even have their own chapter!) KLF2 (I call this guy "KLIFF") is actually *created* by blood flow and shear stress, whereas Nrf2 (aka "Nerf") is *increased* by blood flow and shear stress. Working together, have a "gene profile" of over one thousand genes, meaning they will affect the way those genes are deployed and how they will work to achieve their results. Contrast that with the physician's attempt to treat a condition using a single drug. Sure, he or she might give you a "cocktail" of medicines containing two or three different drugs, but it's nowhere near the complicated and exquisitely balanced "cocktail" your body creates in response to just a little walking.

Walking, thanks to the muscle pump in the legs, is the perfect way to increase circulation, blood flow, and transduction or myokine production. Once the new chemicals (genes, hormones, peptides, etc.) are produced, the circulation delivers them to the cells where they are needed. The body coordinates all the parts and functions of this process like a well choreographed ballet.

A lot of this book will be about walking. There are many books about walking, so why write another? Because the other books tend to concentrate on the *exterior* experiences of walking, and this book wants to tell the "inside, body chemistry story." There is, however, a significant area of overlap and we will explore that in detail.

Am I a doctor or fitness guru? No, I'm an old man, an 83-year-old, with flat feet. I wear arch supports. I have a bunion. I'm not athletic. I have what is generally (and generously) called a "Dad bod." A few years back when I began walking, I had several bouts of plantar fasciitis (inflammation of the bottom of the foot). I have had gout that caused excruciating pain in the joint behind my great toe. So, no, I'm not the sort of person you'd expect to write this book, but I figured that if someone in *my shape* could get into walking, that might encourage you to do it, too.

"I'm convinced that walking is the best all-around form of exercise."

—Dr. Andrew Weil

Start where you are.

Grab some comfortable shoes and start walking. Maybe you will only make it to your neighbor's driveway before you want to turn back. That's fine. You started. Tomorrow, maybe you'll make it past *two* neighbor's driveways. That's progress, and that's success! Two things are of primary importance: you started and you're not quitting. If you think you need to walk thousands of steps to get any benefits, it might seem overwhelming. But that is not the case.

The amount of exercise recommended by all major health organizations is 150 minutes per week of moderate intensity exercise, which includes walking at a brisk pace. This is usually divided into 30 minutes per day for five days. You can further divide it into three ten-minute sessions or even ten three-minute sessions. But remember, walking as little as 30 minutes *a week* is better than zero minutes a week.

A study done in 2020 by researchers in England, Scotland, Canada, Australia, and Denmark discovered that very short periods of physical activity— as little as one or two minutes — resulted in very impressive health benefits. They used wearable devices (like a FitBit) that can capture body movements such as brief bursts of vigorous intermittent lifestyle physical activity that is just a part of everyday life; ordinary things like running after your kids, mowing, climbing stairs, mopping, gardening, doing laundry. They collected data from 25,000 non-exercising men and women with an average age near 60 and followed up for seven years.

Those people who had three bouts per day (lasting one or two min each) showed a 38% to 40% reduction in all-cause and cancer death risk and a 48% to 49% reduction in cardiovascular death risk. Those who recorded activities totaling 4.4 min per day reduced their chances of all-cause death and cancer death by 28%. They also reduced their chances of cardiovascular death by 33%. In 4.4 minutes per day!

The researchers obtained similar results when repeating the above analyses for 62,344 people who exercised. The results indicated that small amounts of vigorous everyday physical activity resulted in substantially lower risk of death.

If you've been thinking, "What is the absolute minimum I have to do to get benefits?" now you know. Remember: *some is good, more is better, everything counts.*

Do you have TEMPA?

There is a Darwinian neuro-physiology and psychology at work in many people that tends to make us minimize physical efforts, commonly called TEMPA, which stands for Theory of Effort Minimization in Physical Activity. No Kidding. This is not just some get-out-of-jail-free card for slackers (not implying that you are one), but it's an actual condition with several peer-reviewed papers examining it in great detail, using many elaborate doctor words.

One 2021 paper from researchers in Canada and Switzerland says:

> "Cues related to sedentary behaviors would be evaluated positively which would contribute to explanations of the physical inactivity pandemic. However, the discrete nature of this approach dichotomizing movement-based behaviors in physical activity on the one hand and sedentary behaviors on the other hand is limiting and prevents an accurate theorization of movement-based behaviors. As supported by the physical and neuroendocrinal adaptations described above, humans have evolved to minimize physical effort throughout the entire energetic continuum."

What all those ten-dollar words (dichotomizing!) mean, is that given a choice between going to the gym or having a donut, *the donut will always win.* Sitting there eating our grease and sugar laden delight, we will feel like a winner, too, but of course, we all know that is far from the truth. Here's another quote from that same paper:

> "In TEMPA, the automatic attraction to physical effort minimization is conceptualized as a neuropsychological process at the level of the individual favoring the implementation and development of cost-effective behaviors. TEMPA posits that movement-related cues are perceived as effortful and that this effort is processed as a cost, that is, an aversive object to be avoided or minimized."

What all this doctor-talk is trying to say, is that we are all internally hard-wired to avoid or minimize exercise. *It's not your fault, it's your genes.*

We're assuming, however, that your reason for buying this book was *not* to avoid exercise. We just wanted to show you how low the threshold is for your entry into a better, healthier future. Here's more good news.

The Benefits of Silly Walking

In 1970, Monty Python aired a skit featuring John Clese as Mr. Teabag, who worked at the Ministry of Silly Walks. In the skit, Clese would walk forward a few steps then take a step backward, then kick one leg high into the air, walk forward a few steps, stagger sideways, walk while half-squatting then repeating the sequence with some variations. A Mr. Putey had a similar although less extreme gait.

Almost unbelievably, the kinesiology (study of movement)

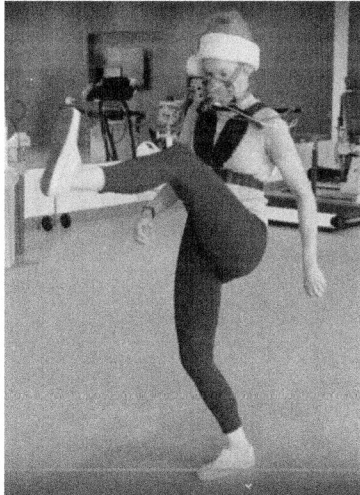

departments of universities in Kansas and Virginia, decided to do a study of inefficient (silly) walking to determine if there were any health benefits to be derived from such walking.

They asked thirteen healthy volunteers (six women, seven men) to perform three 5-minute walking trials around a 30-meter course while wearing a mask to determine their oxygen uptake and energy expenditure (calories burned). The Mr. Putey style of walking raised their oxygen and energy uptake a moderate amount. The Mr. Teabag style of walking raised those figures by 250 percent! The energy required to walk Teabag style, they discovered, places it in the "vigorous" category of exercising rather than the "moderate" category of regular walking. This is the equivalent of jogging. This means that fifteen minutes of daily silly walking per day/5 days per week, (75 minutes total) will equal the recommended 150 minutes of weekly moderate exercise, or 75 minutes of vigorous exercise recommended by all health organizations.

The TEMPA-PEMPA Tango

The authors of the Monty Python Inefficient Walking study proposed a new term, PEMPA- the Practice of Effort Maximization in Physical Activity, in honor of "the unrecognized genius of Monty Python's Ministry of Silly Walks." They really like silly walking. They even surmise that if an initiative to promote silly walking had been adopted in the early 1970's, "we might now be living among a healthier society." The lead investigator has the initials, GAG. Coincidence? I think not.

Here are links to the Monty Python videos:

The original skit:
https://www.youtube.com/watch?v=TNeeovY4qNU&t=110s

The medical study:
https://www.youtube.com/watch?v=FhRLg0IDyhM

If you're the sort of person who is NOT looking for the easier way, perhaps you're looking for the *best*, most *challenging* way, the way that will lead to the *best possible outcome*, then you need to look at Nordic Walking.

Nordic Walking

Walking is an excellent method for exercising your lower extremities and gaining important cardiovascular benefits. Your upper body, on the other hand, receives far fewer benefits. To remedy this situation, there is perhaps nothing better than Nordic Walking. Leena Jaaskelainen, a physical education instructor in Helsinki, Finland, introduced "Walking with ski poles" into her student's lessons in 1966. She recognized the benefits of using the poles while walking. When she joined the faculty of the University of Jyvasyla, she continued teaching walking as physical education and developed a range of exercises with poles.

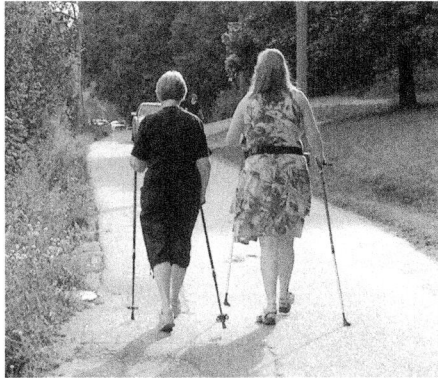

Creative Commons / Wikimedia

As pole walking gained popularity, some early leaders got together with the management team of Exel Oy, a manufacturer of ski poles, among many other industrial products, to develop specialized poles for the new sport. In 1997, Exel Oy came up with several poles and today the company's catalog boasts dozens of different pole designs. https://www.exelsports.com/poles/ Exel also changed the name from "pole walking" to "Nordic Walking."

In 2000, Aki Karihtala founded the International Nordic Walking Association (later renamed a Federation), which began developing educational programs and instructor networks that spread to other countries. There is one in the USA, https://americannordicwalking.com/.

Nordic Walking burns *more calories* and works *more muscles* than conventional walking. Basically, Nordic Walking mimics the motions of cross-country skiing by using poles to push

yourself as you walk along a trail or sidewalk. It was originally used as a summer training routine for cross-country skiers.

Nordic Walking is a common pastime among older adults in Europe. If you go to the train station on Saturdays you'll find droves of people waiting to go up to the mountains to walk with Nordic poles.

Nordic walking combines cardiovascular exercise with a vigorous muscle workout for your shoulders, arms, core, and legs. When you walk without poles, you activate muscles below the waist. When you add Nordic poles, you activate most of the muscles of the upper body as well. You're engaging 80% to 90% of your muscles, as opposed to 50% with regular walking, providing a substantial muscle-building and calorie-burning benefit.

Lots of evidence confirms that Nordic Walking burns more calories than regular walking with estimates ranging from 18% to 67% more. Nordic walking is also associated with reductions in

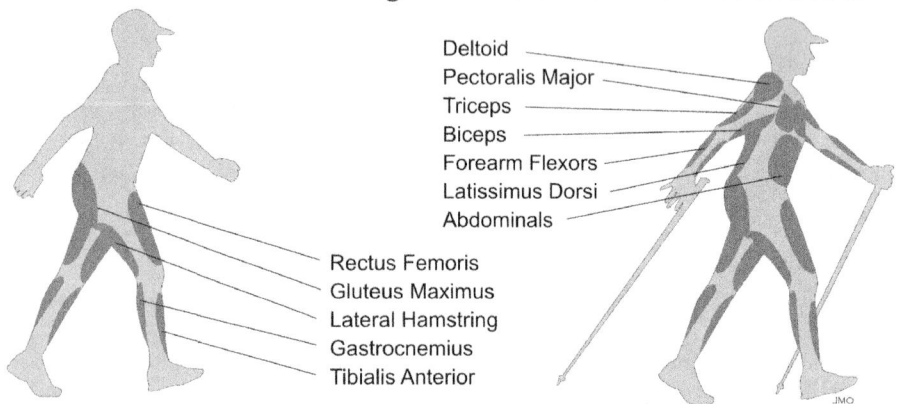

Deltoid
Pectoralis Major
Triceps
Biceps
Forearm Flexors
Latissimus Dorsi
Abdominals

Rectus Femoris
Gluteus Maximus
Lateral Hamstring
Gastrocnemius
Tibialis Anterior

testimonies of reductions in depression, anxiety, chronic pain, and waist circumference. On the other hand, Nordic Walking increases HDL "good" cholesterol, endurance, muscle strength and flexibility, walking distance, cardiovascular fitness, and quality of life. That's quite a boost from those poles!

Other benefits of Nordic Walking include an increase in stability when you use poles, because you have more ground contact points and you're not relying just your two feet. Plus, Nordic walking is fun. It can be a great social activity if you join one of the Nordic Walking clubs popping up across the country. To find one near you, search the Internet or contact your local parks and recreation department or library.

Nordic Walkers are serious about their poles.

Unlike trekking or hiking poles, which have loose straps that go around your wrists, real Nordic poles have a special glove-like system attached to each pole. You slide your hand into it and use your palm rather than your fingers to transmit power to the poles.

Some people maintain that you *cannot* do Nordic Walking without the proper poles. If you go online to do your pole shopping, you'll find that Amazon has 243 listings ranging in price from $20 to $220, and Walmart has 214 similar listings. Almost all of them have a 4.5-star review with little difference in ratings between low- and high-priced poles. Most are collapsible and most are also adjustable in length.

The length is determined by the distance from the ground to your hand while it is extended at a 90 degree angle from the elbow (see illustration).

Let me suggest that if you buy the cheap poles, hold them wrong and use them wrong, you'll still find that your upper body gets a workout. There will be no question that you have upped your fitness game

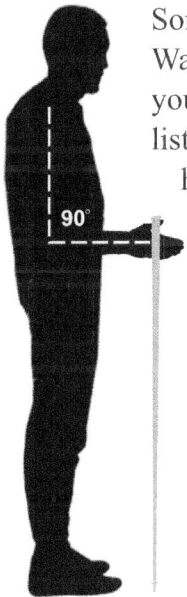

significantly. If you are seriously into fitness, however, I don't doubt the wisdom of acquiring the best tools you can afford.

In addition to good equipment, you will need instruction. This can cost two or three hundred dollars for one-on-one instruction. You may be able to reduce this if you can find group instruction in your area. These people are generally certified by Nordic Walking Federation member organizations.

You will discover that it's not as easy as it seems. I'm a newcomer to Nordic Walking and I intentionally do it on dark nights so that my drunk-camel-on-icy-road version of Nordic Walking is hidden from the neighbors. And yet, I benefit.

There are several Nordic walking techniques. One is "double poling." It involves planting both poles symmetrically in front of you and pulling yourself forward as you walk a few steps. You double pole and then walk three steps. Double pole; one, two, three. Double pole; one, two, three.

Another technique is "single poling," which mimics what our feet are doing, with just one pole in front of you for each stride. Do this either with the same-side arm and leg together or with the opposite arm and leg together. "The pole and foot will always be striking and propelling at the same time. The difference is whether it's on the same side or the opposite side. You're probably going to be more comfortable starting out with single poling, and gradually increasing your speed.

If you have been paying attention, you know that the real benefit of Nordic Walking is increased blood flow and transduction that leads to healthy changes in your body chemistry. With more muscles at work, you're moving more blood and restoring health to your cells, driving mitochondrial biogenesis and antioxidants throughout your body. Give it a try!

From the US and British Nordic Walking websites, I compiled a summary of benefits you can derive from Nordic Walking:

Combines upper and lower body workout for maximum health benefits.

Works all major muscle groups in the body.

Increases oxygen consumption.

Burns up to 46% more calories than regular walking.

Can lead to a 14% reduction in upper body fat.

Strengthens upper body, core, arms, chest, back, buttocks, and legs.

Improves posture and flexibility.

Reduces stress on joints and is low impact.

Suitable for people of all ages and fitness levels.

Ideal choice for improving overall health and wellbeing.

Up to 14% increase in biceps strength.

Reduces waist circumference as much as 8%.

Increases aerobic capacity 8%.

As much as 6% reduction in body mass index.

If you're already walking, the addition of Nordic Poles will not require any more time, just a little more effort that can bring you all these benefits. And I hope you noticed: they don't even mention the incredible cascade of chemical benefits you get through transduction! Think of all the extra muscles now working to make the good chemicals your body needs. The truth is, you already know more than most people do about the blood-flow and transduction-derived benefits of walking!

There are many videos on YouTube about all aspects of Nordic Walking. Your local walking club (if you have one) can help you find instructors and walks where you can participate with a group if you'd like. Here are three videos to help you get started.

https://www.youtube.com/watch?v=MKRrRCUMHOg
For beginners.

https://www.youtube.com/watch?v=zAmsHhc2zCw
Walking movements.

https://www.youtube.com/watch?v=WP2P6tZdmH4
Why walking poles.

"If you are in a bad mood, go for a walk. If you are still in a bad mood, go for another walk."

– Hippocrates

By this point, I hope you're developing a new respect for the act of walking, a seemingly simple and everyday activity, that is actually a powerhouse for our bodies, intricately woven into the fabric of our well-being. In succeeding chapters, we will embark on a journey to unveil the multifaceted ways in which walking serves as a (1) defender, (2) maintainer, and (3) repairer of our physiological systems. We delve into the details, scientific insights and research findings shaping our exploration, shedding light on the profound benefits that walking bestows upon our bodies.

1. Defender Against Chronic Diseases

Walking stands as a formidable shield, offering protection against a myriad of chronic diseases that pose significant threats to our health. Let's explore the robust defenses that walking erects:

Cardiovascular Health

Regular walking plays a pivotal role in cardiovascular health. It enhances circulation, reducing the risk of heart disease and stroke. The rhythmic contraction of muscles during walking aids in blood flow, preventing the buildup of plaque in arteries.

Metabolic Health

Walking acts as a metabolic superhero, fortifying our defenses against diabetes and obesity. It improves insulin sensitivity, helping regulate blood sugar levels, and contributes to weight management.

Mental Well-being

Walking extends its protective embrace to mental health, acting as a defense against stress, anxiety, and depression. It stimulates the release of endorphins, the body's natural mood enhancers.

2. Maintainer in Sustaining Optimal Functionality

Beyond defense, walking assumes the role of a vigilant maintainer, nurturing optimal functionality across various systems within the body:

Joint and Muscle Harmony

Contrary to the misconception that walking might harm joints, it is a key player in maintaining joint health. Weight-bearing exercise, like walking, strengthens muscles and supports joint flexibility.

Spinal Alignment and Posture

Walking contributes to the maintenance of proper spinal

alignment and posture. The rhythmic motion engages core muscles, promoting stability and reducing the risk of back problems.

Cognitive Sustenance, Feeding the Brain

The cognitive benefits of walking extend beyond defense to maintenance. Regular walking has been associated with preserving cognitive function and reducing the risk of cognitive decline in aging populations.

3. Repairer / Healer on Cellular and Physiological Levels

In addition to defense and maintenance, walking emerges as a gentle repairer, promoting healing at cellular and physiological levels.

Brisk walking for seventy-five minutes a week added almost two years to people's life expectancy.
An hour a day added four and a half years.

Nir Barzilai, *Age Later*

Cellular Detoxification:

Walking induces a mild sweating response, facilitating the elimination of toxins from the body. This natural detoxification process aids in the repair and renewal of cells.

Inflammatory Control and Tissue Repair

Chronic inflammation is a precursor to various diseases. Walking helps regulate inflammation through increasing your body's production of anti-inflammatory agents while promoting tissue repair by enhancing blood flow, which delivers nutrients and oxygen to damaged tissues.

Preservation of Bone Density

Weight-bearing activities like walking contribute to bone density preservation. This, in turn, aids in the repair of microdamage within bones, promoting skeletal health.

Walking — your mild-mannered, Clark Kent skill — turns out to be a superhero skill!

The many benefits of walking extend far beyond the realm of mere physical activity. It is a defender, helping us maintain a vigilant stance against chronic diseases. Simultaneously, it assumes the role of a maintainer, nurturing optimal functionality across various physiological systems. Finally, walking emerges as a gentle repairer, facilitating healing on cellular and physiological levels. As we lace up our walking shoes, let us recognize and appreciate the powerful guardian that walking is — a timeless and accessible helper for our well-being. With every step, we journey toward health defense, maintenance, and repair, leading us toward a SuperAger quality of life.

4

Diving Deep With Nerf and Cliff

Two of my favorite molecules I call Nerf and Kliff. Nerf is actually Nrf2[1], and Kliff is KLF2[2]. I doubt that you've ever heard of them, yet they control the majority of changes in your body chemistry that you can influence through your actions. They do a lot of things separately, but many tasks are accomplished when they work in tandem. We will run into them again, but in this chapter, we will be talking about their role in oxidation.

The process of oxidation in the human body can damage cell membranes and other structures, including cellular proteins, lipids (fats) and DNA. What is oxidation? When oxygen is metabolized, it creates unstable molecules called "free radicals," which steal electrons from other molecules, causing damage to DNA and other cells. Here is a picture of oxidation on a steel body of a car. Yes, it's rust, also known as iron oxide.

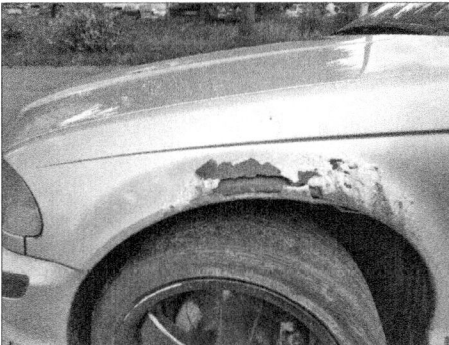

Your body does not rust, of course, but the

effects of oxidation in your body can be just as destructive as rust is to a car. The head of the oxidation gang that's trying to corrupt your body is called superoxide. You could call it a supervillain. This chart shows the far-reaching effects of oxidation.

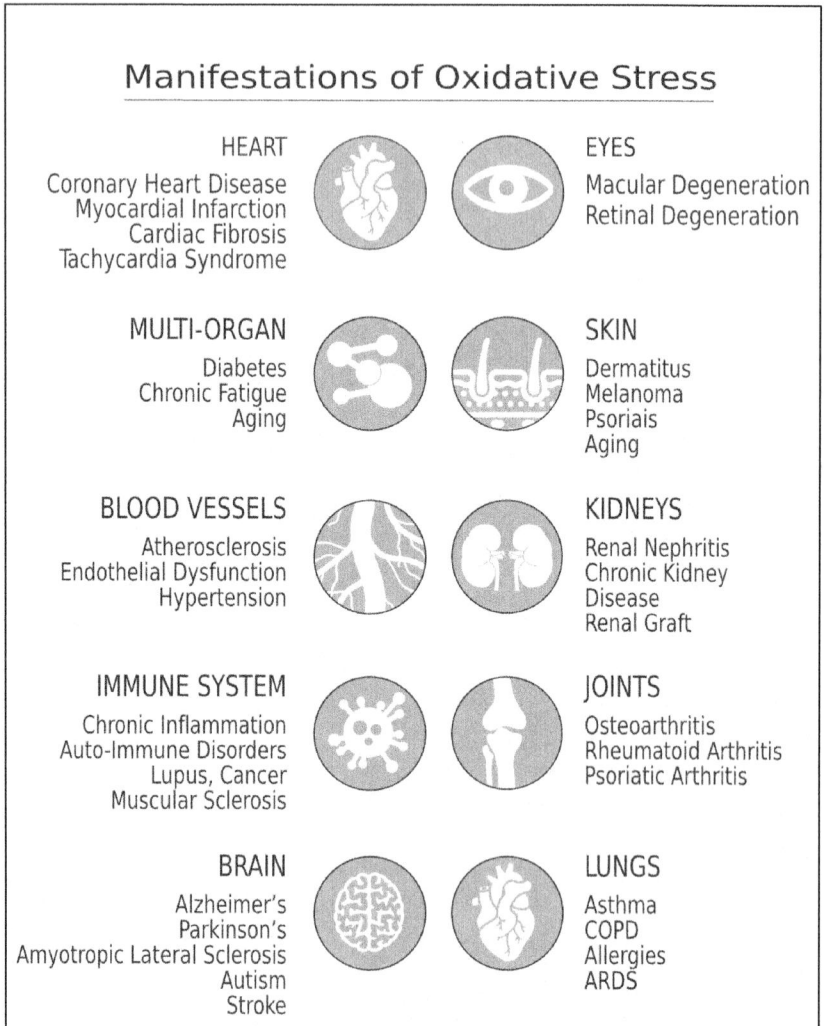

Manifestations of Oxidative Stress

HEART
Coronary Heart Disease
Myocardial Infarction
Cardiac Fibrosis
Tachycardia Syndrome

EYES
Macular Degeneration
Retinal Degeneration

MULTI-ORGAN
Diabetes
Chronic Fatigue
Aging

SKIN
Dermatitus
Melanoma
Psoriais
Aging

BLOOD VESSELS
Atherosclerosis
Endothelial Dysfunction
Hypertension

KIDNEYS
Renal Nephritis
Chronic Kidney
Disease
Renal Graft

IMMUNE SYSTEM
Chronic Inflammation
Auto-Immune Disorders
Lupus, Cancer
Muscular Sclerosis

JOINTS
Osteoarthritis
Rheumatoid Arthritis
Psoriatic Arthritis

BRAIN
Alzheimer's
Parkinson's
Amyotropic Lateral Sclerosis
Autism
Stroke

LUNGS
Asthma
COPD
Allergies
ARDS

That's a lot of really stinky problems to come from one cause, and there are probably a few that we missed. On the other hand, your body has assembled a group of powerful and effective antioxidants (Superheroes?) to combat this dark force. First is SOD[3] that converts superoxide to H_2O_2[4], which is better, but still an oxidant. Two more antioxidants, GPx[5], and CAT[6] work their antioxidant magic by stripping one molecule of oxygen away from the H_2O_2 leaving H_2O – water, and oxygen. Inert. Non-oxidizing. Good stuff.

As mentioned earlier, Kliff and Nerf are good buddies who often work together and their defense against oxidative stress is a perfect example. Kliff is called "flow-dependent" in doctor-talk.

What that means is that if you don't have good blood flow and shear stress, you don't have any Kliff. (A reminder, shear stress is the friction caused by blood rubbing against the lining of blood vessels [the endothelium]. If you're having problems with the term "shear stress", just call it "blood friction". It's like static electricity: no friction, no electricity). Here's an illustration that's sort of complex, but accurately shows how Kliff and Nerf team up to mobilize your inner antioxidant army. *4.2*

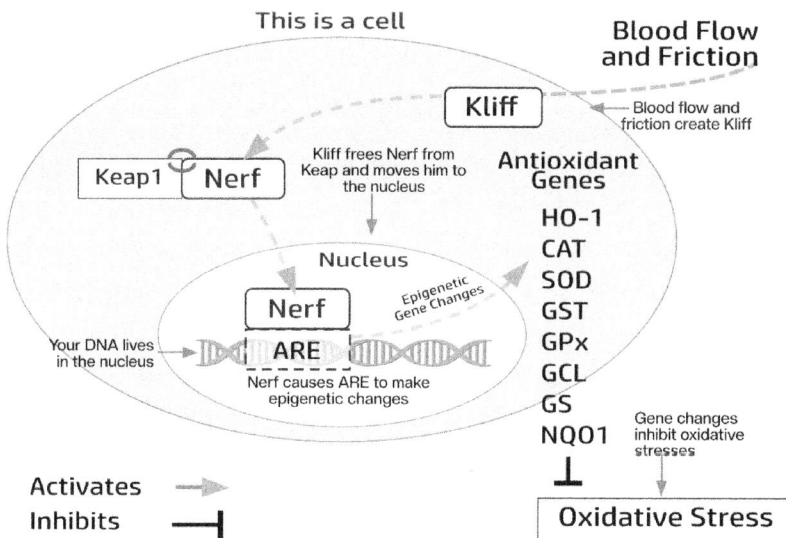

If you walk, play pickleball, dance or whatever, your blood starts moving. The moving blood creates friction on the blood vessel lining (endothelium) bringing Kliff to life. Kliff finds his buddy, Nerf, handcuffed (*negatively regulated* in doctor talk) to something called, appropriately, Keap1, which keeps Nerf from entering the nucleus where he can do some real good for your body. When Kliff sees this, he breaks the handcuffs, grabs Nerf and moves him into the nucleus *(translocates* in doctor talk). Once in the nucleus, Nerf goes to work and finds the ARE (antioxidant response element) segment of your DNA.

Now, things get complicated and really interesting. Your DNA contains the genetic code (your genes) that determines almost everything about you from the color of your eyes, skin, and hair to the shape of your nose to your propensity for certain diseases. Each DNA looks like a ladder that has been twisted. Almost all your cells have DNA and each one, if unfolded, is about six feet long. Since you have 37 trillion cells in your body, and most cells contain 46 DNA. that means you have 10 quadrillion feet of DNA in your body, or about 1.9 trillion miles. That's enough to stretch from the Earth to the moon and back (a mere 238,900 miles) about 4 million times!

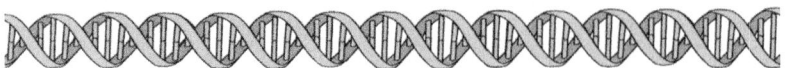

The "rungs" on the ladder are composed of two nucleotides called a base pair. There are about three billion base pairs on each DNA. A gene is a string of DNA that includes anywhere from a few hundred up to more than two million base pairs that encode the information necessary to make a protein. The "code" in your DNA works kind of like the software code that runs your computer. The protein made under the guidance of the code goes on to perform functions in your body.

You inherit half of your genes from your mother, half from your father, and they **never change**. Well, except, sorta, sometimes. It turns out that in addition to your genetics, you have something called **epi**genetics. The "epi" prefix in Greek implies that it is "above" genetics. Epigenetics is a rapidly growing area of science that focuses on the processes that help determine when individual genes are *turned on or off.* While your cell's DNA provides the instruction manual, genes need specific instructions.

In essence, epigenetic processes tell the cell to read specific pages of the instruction manual at distinct times. Most epigenetic changes are temporary, but some changes are stable and can last a lifetime. Some changes can be passed on from one generation to the next, without changing the genes. Here are a couple of examples:

Researchers have discovered that women who are pregnant during stressful times, such as during a war, or as a refugee, or in an abusive marriage tend to have grandchildren who are unusually inclined to be overweight. Women who are pregnant during widespread famine, on the other hand, tend to have grandchildren who are thin. The reasons for "skipping" a generation are not known.

Your "epigenetic switches" can turn specific genes off and on with both immediate and long-term consequences. How do our epigenetic switches get flipped? Through things such as diet, exposure to environmental toxins, smoking, alcohol consumption, stress, and physical activity—*such as walking!* It should be clear to you that you can make epigenetic changes in your own body. For starters, don't eat or drink to excess. Don't smoke. Don't sniff paint or glue. Don't be stupid.

But let's get back to Nerf and his antioxidant trip into the nucleus. He's trying to stop the oxidants from wrecking your body, but there are thousands of genes in your DNA. Where to go? Fortunately, Nerf knows the neighborhood where they all live. It's called the Antioxidant Response Element (ARE) neighborhood and he heads straight to it. Once there, he turns on the antioxidants HO-1, CAT, SOD, and a whole lot more. This means that with the help from our friend NERF, you're fighting off the oxidants and getting healthier. But don't forget, Nerf is there *only* because his friend, Kliff, got him out of those pesky handcuffs and let him into the nucleus. And *who* created Kliff out of thin air by walking, dancing, or gardening? *You did!* Way to go!

Now, don't go overboard with your celebration. If you flop on the couch, eat a family-size bag of jalapeno-onion-butterscotch flavored tortilla chips and wash it down with a 64-ounce mug of root beer, you will kill Kliff and all your good work will be down the drain.

What to tell your friends

Don't tell them about Kliff and Nerf. Tell them you've been studying the molecular biology of blood flow and how it can make epigenetic changes to your DNA that can have profound effects on your oxidative stress levels and overall health. Because that is exactly what you just did! Pretty cool eh?

1. "Nerf" Nrf2 is Nuclear factor erythroid 2-related factor 2
2. "Kliff" is Kruppel-Like Factor 2
3. SOD is Superoxide Dismutase
4. H2O2 is Hydrogen Peroxide
5. HO-1 is Heme Oxidase-1
6. GPx is Glutathione Peroxidase
7. CAT is Catalase
8. DNA is DeoxyriboNucleic Acid

5

Drudgery? No.
It's Me, Me, Meeeee time!

A lot of people faced with the prospect of walking for a long time expect it to be pure unadulterated drudgery. I did, but it's not. There is some of that for sure, but you have so many options and "styles" of walking to make it better. Now, I look forward to it. Sometimes, I will be listening to a program while walking, and if I'm not finished when I reach home, I continue to walk and listen till the end of the program. That can be as much as five to ten minutes later. You've already heard about silly walking and Nordic walking, but how about forest walking, or Mall walking? tai chi walking? Home Depot walking?

Listen while you walk

Listening to music can be a great activity while walking. You can choose your favorite songs or discover new ones from the millions available. Since the optimum pace for walking is 100 steps per minute, you may want to listen to songs that are at that tempo to help with your walk, (think, *Stayin' Alive* by the BeeGees, or *Another One Bites the Dust* by Queen). Check the resources section at the back of the book for a staggering selection of tracks —hip hop, rock, jazz, country pop, classical, yacht rock and more— that are at, or near, the magic 100 beats per minute.

Podcasts have become an increasingly popular form of media, with millions of people listening to them on a regular basis. Listening to a podcast will make the time fly as you're walking. There are many different kinds of podcasts, covering a wide range of topics and genres. Some of the most popular types of podcasts include:

News and politics podcasts: These podcasts cover current events and political issues, often featuring interviews with experts and discussions of current events. Examples include "Joe Rogan," "The Daily," "Pod Save America," "the 7," and "Up First."

True crime podcasts: These podcasts explore real-life crime stories, often delving into the details of high-profile cases. Examples include "My Favorite Murder," "Serial," and "Crime Junkie."

Comedy podcasts: These podcasts are focused on humor and entertainment, often featuring interviews with comedians and other entertainers. Examples include "2 Dope Queens," and "My Brother, My Brother and Me," and "Comedy Bang! Bang!" You can also find a broad assortment of old TV shows online with appearances by Robin Williams, Don Rickles, Gabriel Iglesias, Dave Chappelle, Bill Engvall, Rodney Dangerfield, Jeff Foxworthy, Larry the Cable Guy, Steve Martin, Jonathan Winters, Kevin Hart and so many more.

Science and technology podcasts: These podcasts explore topics such as science, technology, and engineering, often featuring interviews with experts in these fields. Examples include *Radiolab*, "*Scientific American, Houston, We Have a Podcast,* and, from the BBC, *Digital Planet.*

True story podcasts: These podcasts feature real-life stories, often told in a narrative format. Examples include *The*

Moth, This American Life, and *Story Corps.*

Fiction podcasts: These podcasts feature original stories, often told in a serialized format. Examples include "Welcome to Night Vale," "The Black Tapes," and "The Bright Sessions."

Business and self-improvement podcasts: These podcasts offer advice and insights on topics such as entrepreneurship, personal finance, and career development. Examples include *The Tim Ferriss Show, How I Built This,* and *The School of Greatness.* From the Harvard Business Review, there is, *HBR Ideacast,* and Stanford University offers, *Entrepreneurial Thought Leaders.*

Health and wellness podcasts: These podcasts provide information and guidance on topics such as nutrition, fitness, and mental health. My absolute favorite is *Viva Longevity!* With Chris MacAskill. Other examples include *The Mindful Minute, Found My Fitness,* Peter Attia's *The Drive,* Rajsree Nambudripad, MD *The Nutrition Diva,* and *The Rich Roll Podcast,*

Biography. There are a lot from which to choose. Here's a great example: a Polish servant, named Marta, attracted the eye of Peter Romanoff, (Russia's Czar Peter the Great), who married her. She changed her name to Catherine, learned to speak Russian and joined the Russian Orthodox Church, then, upon Peter's death, she became the Czarina and ruled Russia for a couple of years. Her grandson, Peter III, became Czar upon the death of his father. *His* wife (a German named Sophie) changed her name to Catherine, became friends with a few Russian Imperial Soldiers and asked them to "protect" her from her husband who was a drunken oaf. They said, sure, because even though he was their Czar, they didn't like the drunken oaf any better than she did.

Peter abdicated and she became the Czarina, later to become known as Catherine the Great, who apparently turned out to be a pretty good Czarina. I heard the whole story while walking.

Malcolm Gladwell has his own category since he offers a rich buffet of topics that defy narrow classification. He has taught me about Wilt Chamberlain, goiters, iodine, starvation, professional hockey, David and Goliath, containerized shipping, spaghetti sauce, school class sizes, college endowments, the judicial system, and much more.

You can learn a language. Using an app or language learning program to learn and practice new words and phrases while you walk. Some popular language learning apps include Duolingo Babbel, and Rosetta Stone.

You can meditate. Walking can be a great opportunity topractice mindfulness and meditation. Unplug and enjoy the quiet. You can focus on your breathing and the sensations of the world around you. This can help you to release stress, find inner peace and clear your mind. I sometimes walk at daybreak and love to see the dawn start with a glow on the horizon as the birds welcome the day. In the summer, it's the coolest part of the day and is in my opinion, the prettiest part of the day. If the natural sounds of your neighborhood are not pleasant, there are many tracks on youtube with "Meditation Music" which is sometimes mixed with nature sounds such as birds singing, wind and rain, brooks babbling, ocean surf, and "space" sounds.

Some tracks include 40Hz binaural beats, delta brain waves, gamma waves, alpha waves and more. Some of these sites promise better concentration, mental healing, increased brain power, serotonin, dopamine, and financial prosperity. Hmmm,

I'm not sure I believe all this, but I will say that some 40 Hz tracks, listened to for 15 minutes before bedtime, have improved my sleep patterns—I fall asleep quicker and stay asleep longer. How it gets my bladder to go along with this schedule is a mystery to me.

You can listen to an audiobook: Audiobooks can be a great way to pass the time while walking. You can listen to a variety of genres, both fiction and non-fiction. You can learn something new while you walk or be entertained by a captivating story. There are many free sources for audio books, including openculture.com, librivox.org, openlibrary.org, and archive.org. A good place to start is with your local library. In the resources section at the back of this book, you'll find a representative listing of some available books, but it's only the (very small) tip of the iceberg.

Use your walk as an opportunity to plan or organize. Walking can be a great time to think through your day or week, make a mental to-do list, or plan out your schedule. You can use this time to set goals and make plans for how to achieve them. It can be a great way to stay organized and focused.

Don't listen while you walk. It's therapeutic.

A few months ago, I attended a lecture at a local hospital given by a cardiologist who was a member of the American College of Lifestyle Medicine (https://lifestylemedicine.org/). The ACLM is, according to their website, "A society of health professionals united to reverse chronic disease using evidence-based education, practice resources and networking that support the therapeutic use of lifestyle change as the foundation of health and healthcare."

The doctor had treated a patient who had serious cardiovascular problems. A stent was placed, and they put him on a diet that was primarily plant-based. According to his wife, who was in the audience, he is a "big ol,' truck-drivin' county boy," who balked at the diet, but eventually learned to live with it. A few weeks later, however, he returned to the hospital with serious symptoms. When they examined him, however, they found no structural cardiovascular problems and concluded that his problems were entirely caused by stress.

I thought about that for a minute and realized that truck drivers have to deal with schedules, customers, bosses, and worst of all, the endless stream of boneheaded, asleep-at-the-wheel drivers who clog every road in the country. Yep, that's stress.

The doctor prescribed 15 minutes of meditation, daily. Remember, he's a *lifestyle* doctor. As you might suspect, that didn't go over very well with the big ol' truck driver, but, eventually, he worked it out. Since they lived in the country, he would go out into the backyard every morning, sit, and listen. He could hear the birds singing, watch the sunrise, enjoy the cool, fresh country air. It worked. He got better.

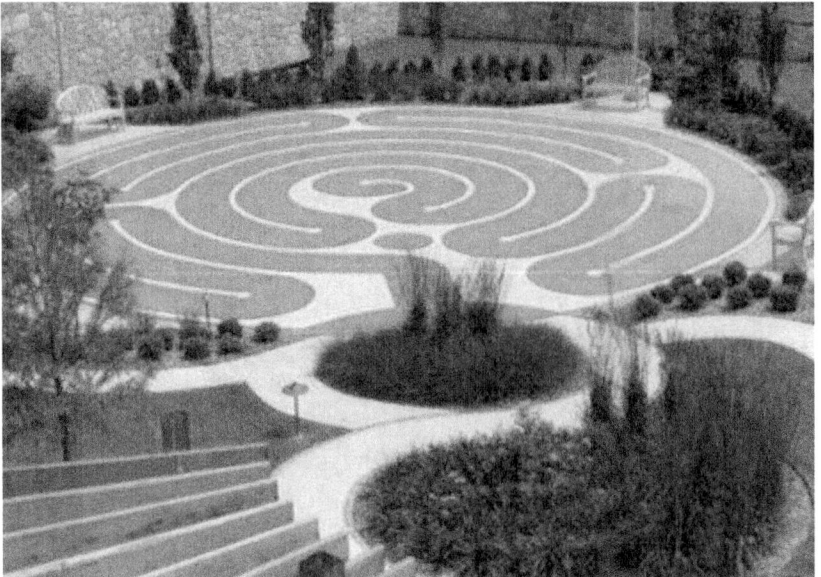

Taking this example to heart, we need to see the value of meditative walking. You may be familiar with labyrinth walking which is used for meditation. It is a single winding path from the outer edge in a circuitous way to the center. Labyrinths are used world-wide as a way to quiet the mind, calm anxieties, recover balance in life, enhance creativity and encourage meditation, insight, self-reflection and stress reduction. Chances are, if you live in a city of any size, there is probably one in your town. In Tulsa there are at least eight, including the one, pictured above, at Phillips Theological Seminary.

Forest walking, or shinrin-yoku, or forest bathing.

Many of us know that taking a walk in a forest is good for us. We can take a break from the noise and pressure of our daily lives. We can enjoy the beauty and peace that envelops you in a natural setting. Strong, peer-reviewed research also shows that forest walking has real health benefits, both mental and physical. Even five minutes around trees or in green spaces may improve your health.

Research shows that walking in forests and parks:

> boosts the immune system
> lowers blood pressure
> reduces stress
> improves mood
> increases ability to focus, even in children with ADHD
> accelerates recovery from surgery or illness
> increases energy level
> improves sleep

Numerous studies in the U.S. and around the world are exploring the health benefits of spending time outside in nature, green spaces, and, specifically, forests. Recognizing those benefits, in 1982, the Japanese Ministry of Agriculture, Forestry and Fisheries even coined a term for it: shinrin-yoku. It means taking in the forest atmosphere or "forest bathing," and the ministry encourages people to visit forests to relieve stress and improve health.

When we are in the forest and we breathe in air, we breathe in phytoncides, which are airborne chemicals that plants give off to protect themselves from insects. Phytoncides have antibacterial and antifungal qualities which help plants fight disease. When we breathe in these chemicals, our bodies respond by increasing the number and activity of a type of white blood cell called natural killer cells or NK. These NK cells kill tumor- and virus-infected cells in our bodies. In one 2010 study, using blood and urine tests, researchers found increased NK activity after a 3-day, 2-night forest trip and the results persisted for more than 30 days afterward.

Walking through trees can also reduce stress levels. Studies show that walking through forests or simply sitting and looking at trees can reduce blood pressure. It can also lower stress-related hormones cortisol and adrenaline. The *Profile of Mood States* (POMS) test evaluates individuals within different mood domains: fatigue-inertia, anger-hostility, vigor-activity, confusion, bewilderment, depression-dejection, tension, anxiety, and friendliness. Using the POMS test, researchers found that forest bathing trips significantly decreased the scores in several of these categories.

If you're among the 85% of the US population that lives in suburban and urban areas, you may not have access to traditional forests. Not a problem. Gardens, parks, and neighborhood trees can serve as an urban or community forest. These green areas are important because they provide your daily access to trees.

Have you ever had to deal with work stress, relationship stress, or the stress of traffic?

Well, of course you have. Who hasn't? And in today's stressful everything-everywhere-all-at-once world it's not getting better. There is a name for how you're feeling. It's called Directed Attention Fatigue.

Some *causes* of Directed Attention Fatigue

Focusing too long on one topic
Fighting, and resisting attractive distractions
Fighting external noise and confusion
Fighting internal noise and confusion
Running ahead in thought
Managing a plan
Monitoring a situation
Attempting to detect deception in others
Attempting to deceive others
Working too much
Getting too little sleep
Dealing with ambiguity

Some *symptoms* of Directed Attention Fatigue include:

Impaired judgment
A "short fuse:" irritability
Failure to notice (or care about) social cues
Restlessness, confusion, forgetfulness
Acting out-of-character
Impulsiveness, recklessness, impaired judgment
Inability to plan or make appropriate decisions
Decreased use of effective thinking tactics and strategies
Degraded problem solving skills

If you have encountered any of this in yourself or others, you know how disruptive this can be in work environments and in families. There are thousands of psychologists and counselors who exist because of this problem. Can walking possibly have an effect on it? Yes, it can! Spending time in nature helps you focus. Trying to focus on many activities or even a single thing for long periods of time can mentally drain us through Directed Attention Fatigue. Spending time in nature, looking at trees, water, birds, and other aspects of nature gives the cognitive portion of our brain a break, allowing you to focus better and renew your ability to be

---

Walking is man's best medicine.

– Hippocrates

If you need peace and healing in your life, *ignore* all the usual advice about walking. *Don't* walk at 100 steps per minute, and *don't* think about your form. Think good thoughts, enjoy the sky, the trees, the birds. Breathe deeply and be thankful. While you may not create as many helpful chemicals through transduction, you will achieve a different kind of health.

If you'd like to learn more about the practice of awe in your life, walking or not, check out the book "Awe: The New Science of Everyday Wonder and How It Can Transform Your Life" by Dacher Keltner

6

Klotho, Named for a Greek Goddess, Is Your Friend

Klotho, was discovered in 1997 by Japanese scientist Makoto Kuro-o and his colleagues when doing research with mice. Their intent was to cause a mutation leading to a different use, but they observed that when they blocked one protein (which they later named Klotho) that the mice died at about 20 percent of the average expected mouse lifespan. They assumed that this indicated a connection with aging, and this led them to inject mice with *additional* Klotho. They were surprised that these mice lived up to 30 percent *longer* than average. Further studies were conducted in mice, and the researchers further discovered that mice lacking the Klotho gene exhibited a range of symptoms resembling premature aging, including shortened lifespan, cognitive decline, shrinking genitals, and vascular calcification.

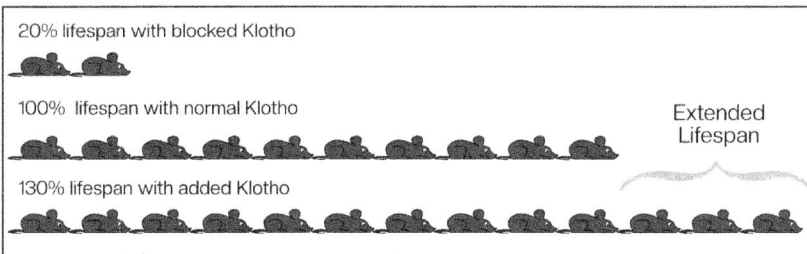

20% lifespan with blocked Klotho

100% lifespan with normal Klotho

Extended Lifespan

130% lifespan with added Klotho

Where does Klotho come from?

Skeletal muscles account for 30–50% of your total body mass and are primarily responsible for locomotion and metabolic homeostasis. In recent decades, it has been discovered that when you contract your muscles, they release various hormone-like substances. These substances are called myokines (myo means muscle, kine means movement), or they are sometimes called exerkines in recognition of the fact that they are secreted by skeletal muscle cells in response to exercise, even moderate exercise—*such as walking!* For a long time, skeletal muscles were only recognized as being involved in the physical movements of exercise. With the discovery of exercise-induced myokines, skeletal muscles have been demonstrated to be involved in the maintenance of homeostasis. Organs that secrete substances are called endocrine organs ("endo" means inside and "crine" means secretes). There are specialists called endocrinologists, who deal with these organs. Calling your muscles an endocrine organ is a relatively new and novel development.

---

scientific reports

Low serum klotho concentration is associated with worse cognition, psychological components of frailty, dependence, and falls in nursing home residents

Begoña Sanz[1,2], Haritz Arrieta[2], Chloe Rezola-Pardo[1,3], Ainhoa Fernández-Atutxa[4], Jon Garin-Balerdi[5], Nagore Arizaga[1,6], Ana Rodriguez-Larrad[1] & Jon Irazusta[1]

Serum alpha-klotho (s-klotho) protein has been linked with lifespan, and low concentrations of s-klotho have been associated with worse physical and cognitive outcomes. Although its significance in aging remains unclear, s-klotho has been proposed as a molecular biomarker of frailty and

---

Klotho Function and Mechanism

The Klotho protein is primarily produced in the kidneys, but it is also found in other organs, including the brain and reproductive tissues. It is secreted into the blood circulation and spinal fluid. It acts as a helper for growth factors and affects several pathways involved in cell growth, calcium, and phosphates. Klotho has anti-aging and tissue-protective effects, and the exact mechanisms are still being studied.

Winning the Klotho lottery

Investigators at UC San Francisco found that people who carry a special variant of the Klotho gene, estimated to be about 20 percent of the population, have more Klotho protein in their blood than non-carriers. Besides increasing the secretion of Klotho in these lucky people, the variant may also change the action of the Klotho protein and is known to lessen age-related cardiovascular disease and to promote longevity.

Let's take a look at the prizes in this lottery:

Klotho Has Anti-Aging Effects: Several studies suggest that Klotho plays a role in extending lifespan and slowing down aging-related processes. There's evidence that higher levels of Klotho can improve cognitive function, reduce age-related cognitive decline, and enhance motor function. The premature death of the Klotho-deficient mice was linked to the development of a syndrome resembling human aging, consisting of premature atherosclerosis (hardening of the arteries), osteoporosis (bone weakness), genital shrinkage and infertility, cognitive disturbances (dementia, Alzheimer's, etc.) and alterations of the hippocampus, which is the part of the brain that handles memory. As shown in the article above, the *lack* of Klotho in our aging population is contributing to a massive decline in the quality of life for our senior citizens. The Klotho deficient mice not only had more sickness and earlier deaths, but they were visibly stunted in growth too, as seen in this photo. *6.3*

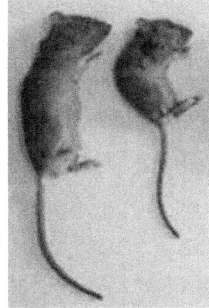

Klotho Improves Kidney Health: The effects of physical activity on aerobic capacity are well known. Unfortunately, Chronic Kidney Disease (CKD) patients present very little tolerance to exercise due to the accumulation of body waste products, obesity, breathing problems, anemia, frailty, and muscle disuse atrophy. All of this leads to lower levels of physical activity compared to the general population. An increase in exercising, if possible, can provide a significant improvement in functional capacity and aerobic capacity. There is a high level of evidence for the improvements that an exercise program brings to functional capacity, with results from the first weeks of exercise.

Klotho has beneficial multi-faceted effects on the kidney. Evidence shows that a decline in serum Klotho level occurs in early chronic kidney disease (CKD) and continues as CKD progresses. Klotho deficiency is associated with poor clinical outcomes and CKD mineral bone disorders. Studies have shown that increasing Klotho levels can protect against kidney damage and slow the progression of renal disease. Klotho supplementation, or exercise-generated Klotho, may have therapeutic value for improving kidney health.

Klotho Improves Cardiovascular Health: According to a research group in Spain, there is evidence that Klotho provides protective effects upon the vascular system such as maintaining of endothelial wall homeostasis and the promotion of vascular health. Klotho can suppress oxidative stress and inflammation, thereby reducing vascular dysfunction. It also offers protection to the cardiovascular system by increasing nitric oxide production. Klotho deficiency, on the other hand, triggers endothelial dysfunction and vascular calcification. Moreover, several clinical studies also suggest that low levels of Klotho are associated with the prevalence and severity of cardiovascular disease and death from all causes. Low Klotho levels are also associated with vascular dysfunction and with atherosclerosis (hardening of the arteries), a common early event in the progression of cardiovascular disease.

Low Klotho levels are a predictor of atherosclerosis (clogged/ hardened arteries), since it is associated with increased fat near the heart, disturbed carotid artery wall thickness and decreased flow-mediated dilation (enlargement of the artery in response to more flow) in healthy subjects. These connections are particularly important in kidney disease patients since most Klotho is generated by the kidneys and it is deficient in people with Chronic Kidney Disease (CKD). A decrease in Klotho levels has been recognized as a risk factor for coronary artery calcification in patients on dialysis. Klotho has been described as a master regulator of cardiovascular disease, with a role in the prevention of atherosclerosis in CKD patients.

The presence of Klotho in your blood is necessary for the proper function of your blood vessels and it protects against the calcification processes. There are many studies that indicate the antioxidative and antiapoptotic (anti-cell death) actions of Klotho. It is also well established that Klotho plays an important role in the prevention of cardiovascular diseases, particularly in the maintaining of appropriate cardiac and vascular function. Klotho is involved in mechanisms of defense against the development of heart hypertrophy (enlargement). There are many studies indicating Klotho deficiency as a factor for cardiovascular diseases. The presence of Klotho in heart cells could be essential for your heart to function, and it may offer protection in some disorders. Given the apparent importance of Klotho, it may be considered an important factor in heart injury, such as myocardial infarction (heart attack). It's more than plausible that Klotho could help protect damaged heart muscle tissue. This opens a new path for the treatment of cardiovascular diseases.

Klotho Improves Cognition: Klotho protein is present in the brain, and it is involved in neuroprotection and cognitive function. Some research indicates that Klotho may protect against cognitive decline, including Alzheimer's disease. However, more studies are needed to fully understand the relationship between Klotho and cognitive health.

Low Klotho levels are associated with a lower score in the psychological component of the Tilburg Frailty Indicator, a worse score in the Coding Wechsler Adult Intelligence Scale, and a lower level of independence activities of daily living. Participants with lower Klotho levels also suffered more falls in the months following their assessment.

Klotho Improves Metabolic Regulation: Klotho protein may be involved in the regulation of metabolic processes, including insulin sensitivity and glucose metabolism. It has been linked to improved insulin signaling and a reduced risk of developing metabolic disorders such as diabetes and obesity.

Klotho reduces frailty and mortality Lower levels of klotho in older adults has been shown to result in increased frailty and all-cause mortality. Physical activity, however, has been shown to increase levels of klotho in the bloodstream, thereby reducing frailty and mortality in the older adult population.

It has been shown that low levels of klotho can lead to premature aging due to hyperphosphatemia (too much phosphate) in mice. In that same study, klotho over-expression extended the average life span between 19% and 31%

Klotho expression declines with age, renal failure, diabetes and neurodegenerative disease. A recent study of American adults showed that low serum Klotho levels correlates with higher rates of death from all causes. Klotho has been recognized for over 30 years as a gene involved in the aging process through its regulation of homeostasis and the activity of fibroblast growth factors.

Increasing levels of Klotho through exercise or supplementation has significant potential as a therapeutic intervention to mitigate loss of physiological function and resilience accompanying old age and to improve outcomes within the disorders and diseases of a patient, viewed as a whole, with special reference to the genetic features of aging. All types of physical activities increased the amount of Klotho, including in postmenopausal women. In a 2021 Japanese study, they found that Klotho was significantly increased in response to a single bout of exercise.

It's important to note that while research on Klotho protein is promising, many studies have been conducted in animal models, and more research is needed to understand its full potential and mechanisms of action in humans.

In addition to walking, increases in Klotho can be accomplished through supplementation of a healthy diet with vitamin D, turmeric, and high protein foods or supplements.

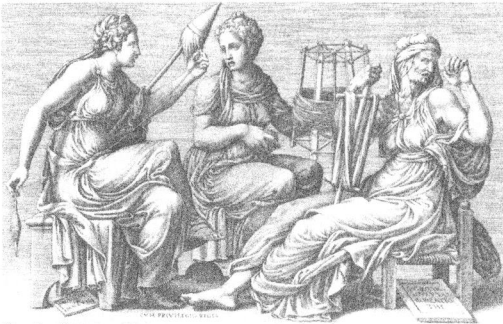

Creative Commons

The three fates of Greek mythology were intended to be personifications of destiny. They were three sisters: Clotho/Klotho (the spinner of the thread of life), Lachesis (the measurer of the thread), and Atropos (the inevitable, who clips it off, a metaphor for death). Atropos looks like she's been visiting the gym too often.

7

If breathing is natural, why do we do such a poor job of it?

Here's the basic function of your lungs: during breathing, oxygen is taken into the lungs, where it passes into the blood and travels to the body's tissues. Carbon dioxide, a waste product made by the body's tissues, is carried to the lungs by blood flow, where it is breathed out. Chances are, you've been breathing for many years without giving it much thought. Actually, we don't *need* to think about it, it just happens. Your diaphragm is a large, thin muscle below your lungs and all of us are born with the knowledge of how to fully engage the diaphragm so we can take deep, belly-filling breaths. As we get older, however, we get out of the habit. Believe it or not, some old men actually "suck in" their stomach attempting to appear slimmer and more attractive. Sure, that will do it.

Unfortunately, many of us gradually shift to shallower, less effective "chest breathing." We fall into this bad habit without being aware of it. This "shallow breathing," where you inhale air into your chest, delivers less oxygen to your lungs and body than the correct "diaphragmatic"

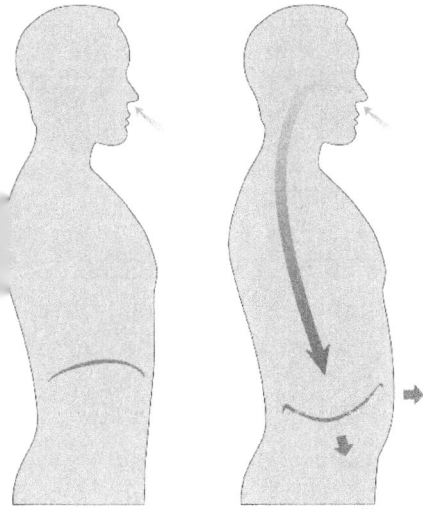

(belly breathing) method. This deeper form of breathing encourages full oxygen exchange — that is, the beneficial trade of incoming oxygen for outgoing carbon dioxide. Not surprisingly, this type of breathing slows the heartbeat and can lower or stabilize your blood pressure. The illustration above shows how the air flows into your body core, and the way your belly, rather than your chest, expands with each breath.

According to Harvard University, here's how to teach yourself to breathe correctly:

Lie on your back on a flat surface (or in bed) with your knees bent. You can use a pillow under your head and your knees for support, if that's more comfortable.

Place one hand on your upper chest and the other on your belly, just below your rib cage.

Breathe in slowly through your nose, letting the air in deeply, towards your lower belly. The hand on your chest should remain still, while the one on your belly should rise.

Tighten your abdominal muscles and let them fall inward as you exhale through pursed lips. The hand on your belly should move down to its original position.

You can also practice this sitting in a chair, with your knees bent and your shoulders, head, and neck relaxed. Practice for five to 10 minutes, several times a day if possible.

"You just put your lips together and blow."

That's a famous line delivered by Lauren Bacall to Humphrey Bogart in the classic 1944 movie, "To Have and Have Not." You can find video clips of it all over YouTube. She's ostensibly telling Humphrey how to whistle, "You know how to whistle, don't you,? You just put your lips together and blow" A few years back, a doctor erroneously gave me a diagnosis of chronic obstructive pulmonary disease (COPD). As a result, I was referred to a physical therapy clinic. One of the first things they had me do was to walk on a treadmill while breathing *in* through my nose and *out* through my mouth with pursed lips. Pursed lips? Oh, you just put your lips together and blow. I get it! Some people say that's what we all do when blowing out candles.

The scientific rationale behind this, as the physical therapists explained to me, is to create back pressure in the lungs so the lung muscles responsible for exhaling will have to work harder. It's sort of like calisthenics for your lung muscles. It makes them stronger. Later, I learned that the back pressure in your lungs also helps to open the air passages in your lungs and more fully eliminate carbon dioxide.

"…daily walking is the closest thing there is to a silver bullet. A magic elixir. A fountain of youth and an all-in-one palliative that that prevents disease, extends life, and improves the quality of that life while we're here".

— Mark Fenton, *The Complete Book of Walking.*

So, if there is a reason to restrict airflow when you *exhale*, how about restricting airflow when you *inhale*? Will that work like calisthenics, too? Yes, it will and there is a peer-reviewed study with all the details.

Daily 'breath training' works as well as medicine to reduce blood pressure.

Simply improving our breathing can significantly lower high blood pressure at any age. Recent research finds that just five to 10 minutes daily of exercises that strengthen the diaphragm and certain other muscles can do that.

Can you believe accumulating evidence indicates that strengthening the muscles you use to *inhale* is beneficial, too? New research shows that a daily dose of muscle training for the diaphragm and other breathing muscles helps promote heart health and reduces high blood pressure. "The muscles we use to breathe can atrophy, just like the rest of our muscles tend to do as we get older," explains researcher Daniel Craighead, an integrative physiologist at the University of Colorado, Boulder, and the lead researcher on the study. To test what happens when these muscles are given a good workout, he and his colleagues recruited healthy volunteers ranging in age from 18 to 82 to try a daily five-minute technique using a resistance-breathing training device which they call. "Inspiratory Muscle Strength Training" (IMST). The hand-held device — there are several on the market — looks like an inhaler combined with a mouth guard, or maybe an adult pacifier. When people inhale through it, the device provides resistance, making it harder to inhale. Sort of the reverse of the "pursed lips" exercise.

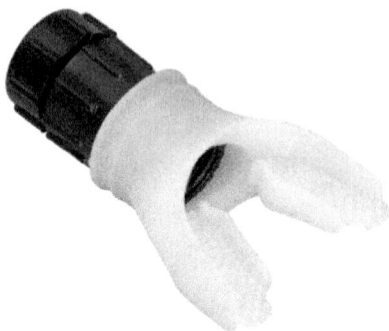

"We found that inhaling 30 times per day for six weeks lowers systolic blood pressure (the first number in your 120/80 or whatever, blood pressure) by about 9, Craighead says. Those reductions are about what you'd expect with conventional aerobic exercise, he says — such as walking, running or cycling.

A normal blood pressure reading is less than about 120/80, according to the Centers for Disease Control and Prevention. These days, some health care professionals diagnose patients with high blood pressure if their average reading is consistently higher than 130/80. The impact of a sustained 9 mmHg reduction in systolic blood pressure is significant, says Michael Joyner, a physician in the study. Before he looked at the results, he'd suspected that young, healthy adults might not benefit as much. "But we saw robust effects," he says, pointing to a significant decline in blood pressure for participants of all ages. He says the finding suggests these IMST breathing exercises could help healthy young people prevent heart disease and the rise in blood pressure that often occurs with aging.

Craighead suspects there may also be benefits for elite cyclists, runners, and other endurance athletes. He cites data that six weeks of IMST increased aerobic exercise tolerance by 12% in middle-aged and older adults. "So, we suspect that IMST consisting of only 30 breaths per day would be very helpful in endurance exercise events," Craighead says. It's a technique that athletes could add to their training regimens. Craighead, whose personal marathon best is 2 hours, 21 minutes, says he has incorporated IMST as part of his own training.

The technique is not intended to replace exercise, he cautions, or to replace medication for people whose blood pressure is so elevated that they're at high risk of having a heart attack or stroke. Instead, Craighead says, "it would be a good additive intervention for people who are doing other healthy lifestyle approaches already."

The Age-Proof Brain, says that "after using the device for five minutes a day for six weeks, participants averaged a 45 percent improvement in vascular endothelial function, while they also showed lower inflammation and improvement in brain function and physical fitness." Impressive results from just five minutes a day!

One of the major obstacles for people in the fitness business is what they call "*compliance*." They give advice to people such as, "Do 30 situps and 30 pushups and run a mile every day," then, they're disappointed that people don't do it. People don't *comply*. But the experts think people are more likely to suck on a plastic thingy five minutes a day. Better "compliance". But here's the kicker. It's not as easy as you might think. After 30 breaths you feel like you've been *exercising*. Oh, wait, that's the point! At least, in my experience. That might be how you'll feel if you're an old man.

Get your buzz on!

A group of researchers at the Karolinska Institute in Sweden and Fredrico University in Italy discovered that the mucosa lining your nose and sinuses releases nitric oxide that can be measured in nasally exhaled air. Your sinuses can produce a large amount of nitric oxide. The study reported that levels of exhaled nasal nitric oxide increased dramatically if a person hums while exhaling rather than exhaling silently. This is most likely due to an increase in nasal sinus vibration caused by the oscillating sound waves. The measured output of nasal nitric oxide increased 700% during humming, which greatly speeds up the exchange of air between the sinuses and the nasal cavity. The high level of nitric oxide that accumulates in the sinuses passes quickly into the lungs where it helps the body in many ways.

We have mentioned Nitric Oxide (NO) before, and it will appear again because it's just that important. NO has many roles in the body, the most important being its protective role in supporting endothelial function and preventing cardiovascular disease. It also is antifungal, antiviral and antibacterial; it supports the brain and neuronal communications; is responsible for vasodilation, glucose uptake, and activation of muscle mito-chondrial energy use.

Within the vasculature, NO induces vasodilation, inhibits platelet aggregation (sticking together in lumps), prevents platelet adhesion to endothelial cells, inhibits smooth muscle cell proliferation, regulates programmed cell death (apoptosis), and helps maintain endothelial cell barrier function (helps it not leak). It is a signaling neurotransmitter and an antimicrobial agent. So, if humming can increase it, *let's hum!*

The Yoga folks have been doing it for centuries!

The Bhramari Pranayama was first mentioned in print during the 14th century. Bhramari means "big black bee." Prana refers to life energy, and yama means to control. It is often referred to as "Humming Bee Breath."

These people are *very* serious about their breathing. And their bees. You can find all kinds of stories about bee breathing on the web as well as videos that demonstrate the proper way to do it. There's even a book about it.

First, you place the thumbs of both hands on the little flaps

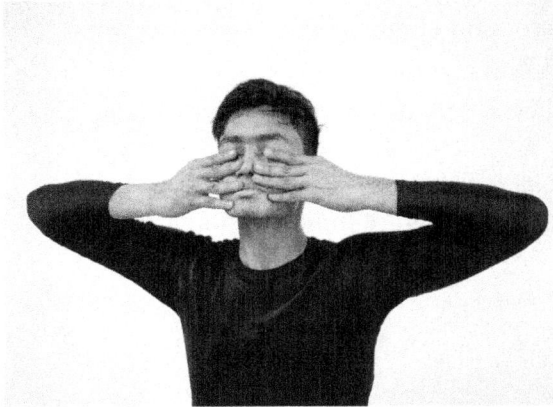

Creative Commons - CC0

near the center of your ears (tragus in Doctor Talk) to block your hearing. Then you place your index fingers on your face above your eyes. The second fingers will go on either side of your nose. The third fingers will be placed between the nose and the lips. Your little fingers will be placed below your lips.

Once in position, you inhale slowly and deeply then slowly exhale through your nose while making a humming sound. Apparently, the pitch is not important, just whatever feels comfortable. You may be surprised at how *loud* it is in your head. It reminded me of using an oscillating sander on a sheet of plywood in a small garage.

One website that I visited describes a pretty sophisticated process that comes from the humming bee breathing technique:

"Bhramari pranayama requires an audible humming sound. This, of course, requires the vocal cords to vibrate. And because a branch of the vagus nerve innervates the vocal cords, vocalizations (such as humming) stimulate the vagus nerve.

The vagus nerve is the longest cranial nerve in the body and it is intimately related to the para-sympathetic nervous system because it has many parasympathetic fibers. By stimulating the vagus nerve, we can help to initiate what is known as the relaxation response.

The relaxation response shifts our body into the parasympathetic nervous system so that we may rest, digest, feed, and breed—ultimately, moving us into states of deeper and deeper calm relaxation."

I'm not sure that I will believe all that, but I *do* believe in the power of nitric oxide to positively affect your body, *so let's hum!* The chart shows the dramatic increase in NO that is the result of humming while exhaling.

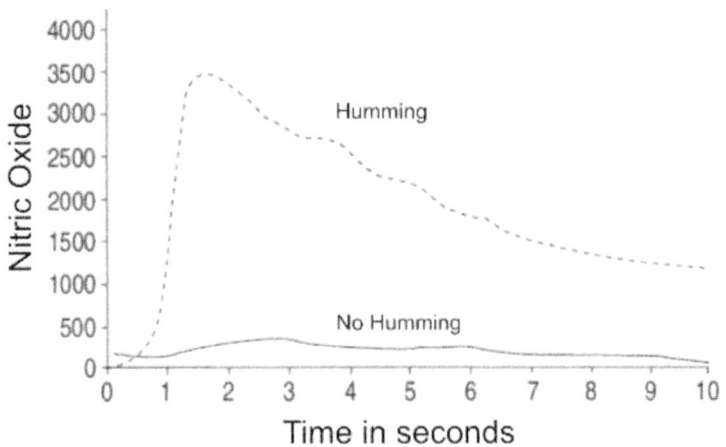

To avoid any liability from things you might do, let me point out that you probably shouldn't try the fingers-over-the-eyes-humming-bee-breathing-technique while walking. Just sayin'.

You might avoid a face-plant experience. On the other hand, I would guess that occasionally using a few humming exhales while walking with your eyes and ears open, may be of benefit to you. I tried humming a tune, and it's less boring.

Don't kill your bacterial friends!

This isn't about breathing, but it's important. While we're talking about all the ways we can boost nitric oxide, we need to point out a big mistake that many of you are making. We have already talked about the way that your body makes NO through blood friction and transduction. But there's another way – it's with food. Eating certain foods will boost your production of NO and the best thing you can eat for that is *green leafy vegetables*. (Wouldn't you just know it!) Here's the problem: These veggies contain **nitrates** which are building blocks for NO, but they have to be turned into **nitrites** before they can travel down your gullet to your stomach and become NO. What turns nitrates into nitrites? *Bacteria that live in your mouth!* Bacterial species with names like actinomyces, corynebacterium, haemophilus, kingella, rothia, and veillonella express an enzyme responsible for the conversion of nitrate to nitrite. Despite their strange and slightly scary names, these guys are your friends. They're called commensal bacteria. Without them you can't live.

If you know the old saying, "An apple a day keeps the doctor away," you might be surprised to learn that the average apple contains 100,000,000 bacteria. That's right, One. Hundred. Million. Bacteria. A cup of yogurt contains a billion or more. But these are good guys. They help the body function properly and when we hurt them, it hurts *us*! Actually, you have around 37 trillion cells in your body, but you have around 39 trillion bacteria, so you're outnumbered!

Obviously, breathing is important to walkers and this section covers a lot of ground in a few paragraphs. If you want to learn more about breathing, check the resources section at the back of the book for information explaining why you should *not* engage in mouth-breathing. If you Google *mouth breathing* you get millions of sites, all of them saying, "don't do it."

You'll also find a nice tutorial on breathing exercises from the Sloan Kettering Cancer Institute. Lastly, you will find an abundance of resources on the internet to learn more. Some are good, some are not. Sometimes it's hard to tell. Be careful what you believe.

8

Explanation of Medical Trials in People-Talk

As mentioned before, much of the information in this book is derived from peer-reviewed articles. It's probable that you don't know what that means (most people don't) and that these articles are usually derived from medical trials (studies) and laboratory experiments. Many, possibly most, people don't know how medical trials are done.

Imagine a terrible new disease in which people have skin that turns purple with green bumps, they smell like snickerdoodle cookies, and they laugh out loud all the time. It's the dreaded LOL disease. Now suppose your friend, Ralph, invents a pill to cure it. You find 100 hospitals, and each has ten patients with LOL. They are given Ralph's pills by hospital staff and then, two weeks later, you call in medical experts to see how it worked. Each of the 1,000 patients is examined by an MD, a DO, a PhD, a PA, a RN, a JD, and your aunt Louise. They all agree that all the patients are 100% healed. You expect this result to be greeted by the medical community and news media with trumpets and loud hallelujahs, right? You're anticipating a call from the Nobel Prize committee. Nope. Not at all. This is the weakest kind of study. It gets no respect. Aunt Louise is fit to be tied.

This is a retrospective (after the fact), observational (the experts are just looking at the evidence), anecdotal (it doesn't have a control arm or randomization, or lots of other stuff) study. It can only show correlation (they took the pill then got well, but it might not have anything to do with the pill), not causality (yep, the pill caused them to get better). If you want respect in the medical community, you must jump through all kinds of quality-enhancing hoops. This is a good thing.

First, a quality trial must be *prospective*, meaning that the principal investigator (PI, but not like Magnum) and his/her investigative team will design the study in advance, detailing all facets of the study including target outcomes and goals.

Next, the investigative team will come up with a *research question*. Something like, "Does Ralph's Magic Pill really affect people with LOL?"

Next, they will decide their *inclusion and exclusion criteria*, such as "The study will exclude people who have naturally purple skin," or "the study will exclude bald people, or people under 18, people with cancer, or whatever." Inclusion criteria might include such things as "The study will include people who are age, sex and race matched to the general population."

Next, the study grows arms. First they have the arm that is getting the real thing (the **experimental arm**), then they will have one or more arms (**the control arm**) which will include placebo (fake) medications or procedures. They might decide to have arms to explore alternatives (different dosages or combinations, etc.). This is done so the investigative team can compare the effects of the new pill against something else to better measure its effectiveness.

Next, they will need to distribute patients among the arms, but first, it is important that they are *randomized*, which is more complicated than you think. Pulling names from a hat? Flipping a coin? Those are certainly random but are never used. The four main types used are:

Simple Randomization
Block Randomization
Stratified Randomization
Covariate Adaptive Randomization

The explanation of these is very complicated and goes on and on. The message here is that they are very thorough in their efforts to eliminate bias and untrustworthy data from the trial.

After randomization, they will need to decide on **blinding**. In a **single-blinded** trial, the *patients* don't know if they're getting a placebo or the real medicine. In a **double-blinded** trial the *patients nor the caregivers* know if they're getting a placebo or the real thing. In a **triple-blinded** trial the *patients, caregivers and even the investigators* don't know which is real or placebo. A third party holds the secret key to that question. The purpose of all this blinding is to avoid the possibility that someone in the investigative team may try to influence the outcome. All this blinding mitigates the possibility of personal bias affecting the outcomes.

So, after designing the study, the investigative team is nearly ready to enroll some patients, but they can enroll them only **after** they are given an **Informed Consent Form**. They, the patient or legally responsible person, must read and understand it before signing. This form must be written in plain, eighth-grade-level English. No big fancy, confusing words. The investigative team is not allowed to put anything in the agreement which will limit their, or their institution's liability. The investigative team is obligated to tell them of any possible bad stuff that can happen to them without minimizing the risks. They must also be given the option of dropping out of the study at any time.

Once your package is put together, you submit it to the *Institutional Review Board* (IRB). This is a group of highly qualified researchers working on behalf of the institution that is doing the research. They can question all aspects of your study and suggest (or mandate) changes. They might question your overall objectives, your methods, your progress milestones, the ethnic makeup of your cohorts, or anything else. You will probably go through a process of making changes and arguing some you don't want to change. Eventually, if you're doing your homework, the study is approved.

Medical trials are called Phase 1, Phase 2, and Phase 3. They start out with one or two dozen people in Phase 1 trials. Phase 2 gets around 50 to 100 people. Phase 3 trials, the kind of study where you get to put your new pharma miracle on the market, can include from 1,000 to 30,000 people or more.

How much do these trials cost? A phase 1 study with 10 people can cost 350 to 500 thousand dollars. Phase 2 will easily cross the low millions mark, and a Phase 3 trial can cost hundreds of millions of dollars. Around half of all Phase 3 trials end up with a drug that is **not** approved for use.

If the investigative team wants to add power and believability to the study, they will conduct the study at multiple locations simultaneously, this is called a **multi-center trial.** This reduces the possibility of bias, ensures a more statistically powerful test, and costs a lot more, of course.

So, let's review. The best trials are:
Prospective, Randomized, Controlled,
Blinded, Multi-center Trials.

The investigative team completes the study and then **collects the data**. The data collected includes administrative and demographic information, diagnosis, treatment, prescription drugs, laboratory tests, physiologic monitoring data, hospitalization, patient insurance, etc. The data collected is generally posted on ClinicalTrials.gov, a registry and results database of privately and publicly funded clinical studies conducted around the world. This resource is provided by the U.S. National Library of Medicine. Each study record includes a summary of the study protocol.

Once the data is in hand, they call in the **Medical Statisticians** who will massage the data into a cohesive bank of data which the investigator team can then analyze and draw their conclusions. They will contrast the actual outcomes against their target outcomes and try to measure the efficacy of the drug or procedure being tested. In this case it's Ralph's Magic pill which seems to have cured 100% of the patients. NOW they will bring in the trumpets and media to celebrate the miracle, right? Nope. The investigative team must first write an article and submit it to a peer-reviewed journal. After it is published, some of the media may write something about it.

As part of their submission, the authors must list all **possible conflicts of interest**, such as serving on the board of a pharma company or being paid to make talks on behalf of a company, or owning stock in medical-related companies. The investigator team members who are given the task of writing the article will try to get the article into the most prestigious publication possible. Journals like the *New England Journal of Medicine*, the *Journal of the American Medical Association*, or *Lancet*, will make your article a winner. Publication in the Journal of the Hooterville Medical Association will sink your boat to irretrievable depths.

When the authors send their article to a journal, the publication will select one or several of their peers to review the paper. These peers are credentialed professionals in a related area of study who have participated in controlled trials and have published articles in other peer-reviewed journals. These reviewers are not identified to your team. They will send their anonymous comments to the authors who can respond if they are asked for more information, or a different perspective, or the reviewers might question some of the study's results and the team must respond. The reviewers can accept, accept with changes or reject the article. This is like running up Heartbreak Hill at the end of a marathon. Very stressful.

If the article gets thumbs up from the reviewers and the publishers, the article will be published. So, *now*, will you get the trumpets and all the rest? Probably not.

Your investigators and authors will **not** write a study article titled, "Miracle Pill Cures the Scourge of the Ages!!! No, they will title it something like, "Combination of stiglerstat and vianical dimethene appears to possibly mitigate some symptoms of LOL. Further studies are warranted." Because that's doctor talk for Wowie! and Gee Whiz!

What does all this have to do with walking?

A lot if you're talking about believable facts. When you're reading an amazing fact and you see a footnote directing you to an article in PubMed, you need to know what it took for that particular fact to be there. Many highly educated people joined their collective expertise and worked their way through an institutional review, then a complex set of high requirements and many safeguards designed for unbiased accuracy of results. The accuracy and adequacy of the story were checked *again* by their peers before it made its way into print. This is a rigorous and thorough process that should give you confidence in the results.

This doesn't mean that all research is error-free, but it certainly keeps to a minimum the possibility that you will be misled. And then there's the grass-roots final check. It's all those peers out there.

If a person, or team publishes a paper that is flawed or fraudulent, it won't be long before other teams of investigators will start to issue their *own* studies saying, "we were **unable to replicate** these results." This is a doctor-talk phrase that means, "we think those guys are either mistaken or they are lying." It is not unusual for articles to attract criticism from fellow investigators. Sometimes, after criticism, the articles are modified, sometimes they are retracted by the investigators, and sometimes they are retracted by the publication. If the criticism alleges fraud, there may be an investigation by professional oversight organizations and/or governmental entities.

There are some people who have low opinions of the medical profession, the government (any country) and pharmaceutical companies. They believe that when a scientist makes a mistake and, subsequently, a pharmaceutical company releases a flawed medication to the market, that a secret network of doctors, researchers, government officials and pharmaceutical people will all work together to keep the truth from being revealed to the public. I don't believe it.

There is a substance, for example, called aldose reductase that plays an important role in how your body processes sugar. If it can be blocked, it will help prevent most of the complications of diabetes. Over the last three decades, more than 100 patents have been issued for aldose reductase blockers. The patent holders are major pharmaceutical firms and major universities around the world. A few have gone through the complete three phase approval process (which, you'll remember, costs hundreds of millions of dollars), yet **not one** has been approved for use in the US. The medical profession and the FDA are not rubber stamps for big pharma and big money. The process is not perfect by any means, but it mostly does what we need for it to do.

9

Brainwalking for Better Cognition

Neurons are the fundamental units of the nervous system, responsible for transmitting and processing information. Neurons consist of a cell body, dendrites, and an axon. The cell body contains the nucleus and other organelles necessary for cellular function. Dendrites are specialized extensions that receive incoming signals from other neurons or sensory receptors. The axon is a long, slender projection that conducts electrical impulses, known as action potentials, away from the cell body toward other neurons, muscles, or glands.

Neurons communicate with each other at specialized junctions called synapses. When an action potential reaches the axon terminal of one neuron, it triggers the release of neurotransmitter molecules (tiny droplets of liquid chemicals) into the synaptic spaces. These neurotransmitters attach to receptors on the dendrites or cell body of the next neuron, generating a new electrical signal. Neurons are the building blocks of the nervous system, forming complex communication networks that underlie all aspects of brain function and behavior.

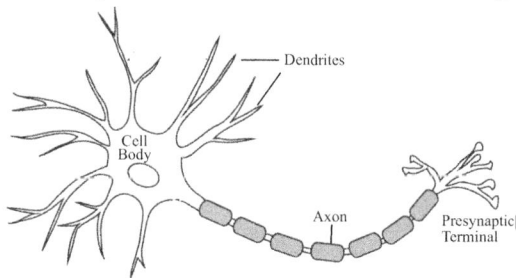

Dendrites

Cell Body

Axon

Presynaptic Terminal

In chapter one with the twins story, we touched on the link between walking and cognitive decline. The link is totally chemical. Your endothelial cells, responding to the friction of blood flow produce chemicals. What kinds of chemicals? Many helpful substances that can impact your brain such as antioxidants, anti-inflammatories, and anti-coagulants. Walking also causes the muscles to produce hundreds of myokines, which are small messenger proteins, that can help block or reduce many of the chemicals that affect your brain, including tau and amyloid beta that contribute to Alzheimer's Disease and Parkinson's Disease.

But, before we go further, let's get a clearer understanding of what cognition is and how it declines with age. Cognitive impairment pertains to challenges or deficits in cognitive functions, which encompass various mental processes such as:

Memory -*the capacity to retain and retrieve information*

Attention -*the ability to concentrate on specific tasks or stimuli*

Executive function -*high level processes such as planning, organizing, or decision making*

Language -*comprehension, expression, and communication through spoken and written language*

Perception -interpreting and comprehending sensory information from the environment

Spatial navigation -*the ability to perceive and navigate the physical space surrounding us*

People who have cognitive impairment, can be classified into various levels from normal cognitive function to mild, moderate, and severely impaired. A person's classification is usually determined by some sort of assessment tool, such as the Mini-Mental State Examination or the American Geriatrics Society criteria. *Mild impairment* includes difficulty with memory, language, visual-spatial skills, and executive function. *Moderate impairment* includes a more significant decline in cognitive abilities which can adversely affect a person's life. They may require assistance in their daily acts of living. *Severe impairment* includes a marked decline in cognitive abilities, leaving an individual unable to perform many daily tasks.

Several factors collectively contribute to the prevalence of cognitive impairment. Some of these factors have a direct impact on cognitive function, while others influence the prevalence of cognitive disorders through their effects on health and lifestyle. Some factors are:

1. Genetics

2. Ethnicity

3. Geographical location

4. Physical activities

5. Gender

6. Nutrition

7. Metabolic diseases

Some of these factors cannot be changed such as your genetics, ethnicity or gender. But the *one item you can change*, physical activities, *can have a profound effect on your cognitive function* as you age.

NOTE: There are lots of chemicals mentioned in this chapter. It is NOT NECESSARY that you know what they are as long as you get a general idea of what is going on. Just skip over them.
Or, give them your own nicknames, like I do!

"The act of walking transcends mere physical activity; it is a potent modulator of brain function and mental health."
A. Dietrich, W.F. McDaniel, 2004

I'm sure it's clear to you by now, that *walking is surprisingly good for your brain.* It raises blood flow which triggers transduction resulting in chemical changes that are beneficial for brain health. Walking affects your brain in at least eleven different ways. We will explain each one of them. Lastly, we will explain the beautifully complex processes that make everything work, along with an illustration that may help clarify everything.

Walking helps protect and preserve cognition in at least eleven ways

In chapter four, we talked briefly about **myokines**, which are proteins acting as hormones and cytokines, secreted by muscles as they contract that make chemical changes to your blood. Walking is an exercise that causes the production of myokines resulting in:

1. The creation of new brain cells
2. Reduction of brain cell death
3. Improved mitochondrial function
4. Reduced oxidative stress
5. Increased autophagy (recycling of old, dying cells)
6. Reduction of inflammation
7. Reduced amyloid beta production (contributes to Alzheimer's disease)

8. Reduced tau (rhymes with cow) production (contributes to Alzheimer's disease)

9. Reduction in stress hormones

10. Improvement in sleep quality

11. Improved mood and cognitive function

New brain cells are created (neurogenesis in doctor talk) when the increased blood flow causes a corresponding increase in the production of Brain Derived Neurotrophic Factor (BDNF). In the US, neutotrophic is pronounced new-row-TRAW-fik, the rest of the world pronounces it new-row-TRO-fik. Some people say nyoo-row. Neurotrophic factors are a family of molecules that support the growth and survival of brain cells.

The hippocampus is particularly responsive to the effects of aerobic exercise. New neurons integrate into existing brain circuits, enhancing cognitive flexibility and memory formation. This process is vital for learning new information and adapting to new situations, underpinning the cognitive benefits of walking and increased blood flow. Another chemical produced is CX3CL1[1]. These two chemicals enable a neural stem cell (a sort of baby cell that hasn't decided what it wants to be when it grows up) and guide its development into a brain cell.

Other neurotrophic factors influenced by walking are vascular endothelial growth factor (VEGF) and insulin-like growth factor 1 (IGF-1). VEGF is pivotal for blood vessel growth, ensuring that increased neural activity is matched with sufficient blood supply. IGF-1 is involved with neurogenesis and synaptic plasticity, facilitating learning and memory processes.

Reduction of brain cell death is accomplished through the combined efforts of five myokines (Apelin, IGF-1[2], FGF2[3], FGF21[4], and LIF[5]) that are like a "pharmaceutical cocktail" that can stop apoptosis (cell death).

Improved mitochondrial function is helped through an increase in Fibroblast Growth Factor 21. You may remember from chapter one where we talked about the mitochondria producing ATP, the fuel (energy) that your body runs on. While it only represents 2 percent of the body mass of the average adult human, the brain consumes an estimated 20 percent of the body's energy supply. Obviously, keeping your mitochondria happy will help sustain your brain power.

Reduction of oxidative stress confers protection against a wide variety of diseases as illustrated in chapter four. Walking-induced blood flow and transduction can bring about increases in many of the body's strongest antioxidants (SOD[6], HO-1[7], CAT[8], GST[9], GPx[10], GCL[11], GS[12], and NQO1[13,] etc.).

Increased autophagy. Autophagy is a natural process by which a cell breaks down old, damaged, unnecessary, or dysfunctional components within a cell and then repurposes those components for fuel and to build or maintain cells. Autophagy is important as these "junk" components take up a lot of room in a cell and can prevent it from working properly. Autophagy also destroys disease-causing pathogens, such as bacteria and viruses, that can harm cells.

"Auto" means self and "phagy" means eat. So, the literal meaning of autophagy is "self-eating." This is basically one of the body's processes to "take out the trash." As people age, their autophagy processes slow down. Some people feel that this contributes to the aging process that ends with mortality. Autophagy in mitochondria is sometimes called mitophagy.

Reduction of inflammation. Inflammation is the immune system's response to harmful stimuli such as pathogens, damaged cells, toxic compounds, or irradiation. Inflammation acts by removing injurious stimuli and initiating the healing process —it is, therefore, a defense mechanism that is vital to health. When it becomes chronic, however, it is destructive to the body. Neuroinflammation (brain cell inflammation) affects certain brain cells. Walking-induced blood flow increases levels of six anti-inflammatory chemicals (Apelin, FGF2[3], FGF21[4], IGF-1[2], Irisin[14], and CX3CL1[1]) which serve to block or reduce inflammation in brain cells.

Reduced amyloid beta and tau production. These substances are commonly known as "tangles" and "plaques" that can interfere with the transmission of signals between nerve cells as shown in the illustration. When a message is transmitted from your foot, for example, it passes through a *series* of nerves. There is not one long nerve that delivers the message to your brain. Every few millimeters or inches the message must jump from one nerve cell to another across a gap called a synapse.

How messages travel through nerves

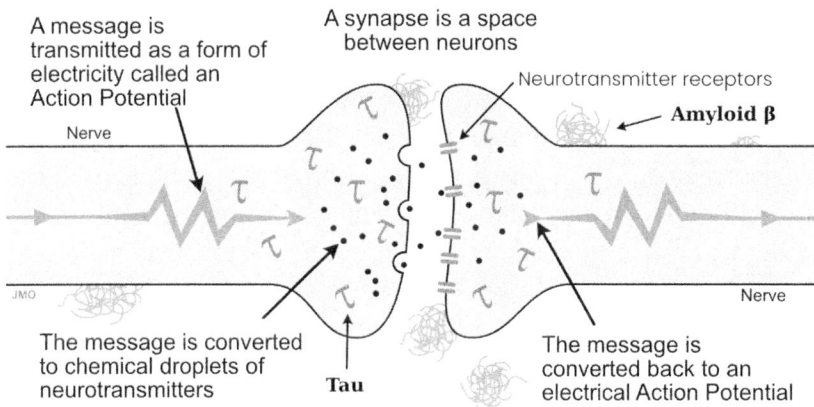

A message is transmitted as a form of electricity called an Action Potential

Nerve

A synapse is a space between neurons

Neurotransmitter receptors

Amyloid β

The message is converted to chemical droplets of neurotransmitters

Tau

The message is converted back to an electrical Action Potential

Nerve

JMO

The electrical message is transformed into tiny droplets of neurotransmitters that jump across the synapse to be caught by receptors on the next nerve and continue its journey to the brain. These chemicals fit into their receptors like a key into a lock. Both tau and amyloid beta in and around the synapse can "gum up the works," creating havoc in the delivery of messages. It is broadly believed that they contribute to the problems of Alzheimer's disease. Walking-induced blood flow increases levels of chemicals (BDNF, FGF2[3], IGF-1[2], CX3CL1[1], and FGF21[4]) which have been shown to reduce or block both amyloid beta and tau.

Reduction in Stress Hormones. Walking reduces levels of the body's stress hormones, such as adrenaline and cortisol.
Regular walking moderates the hypothalamic-pituitary-adrenal (HPA) axis, responsible for stress response regulation. Diminishing the secretion of cortisol and adrenaline helps mitigate the adverse effects of chronic stress on the brain, including the potential reduction in hippocampal volume, which is associated with memory and mood disorders.

Improvement in Sleep Quality. Regular walkers often experience improvements in sleep quality, which is directly linked to better cognitive function and mental health. Good sleep helps consolidate memory and repair neuronal damage, reducing the risk of cognitive decline.

Improved sleep quality and efficiency following regular physical activity are thought to result from physical tiredness and the normalization of sleep phases. Moreover, exercise-induced reductions in anxiety and depression contribute to better sleep patterns, creating a virtuous cycle of sleep and exercise benefiting mental and cognitive health.

Improved Mood and Cognitive Function The physical activity of walking can improve mood and cognitive function by increasing the production of endorphins and endocannabinoids—chemicals in the brain that act as natural painkillers and mood elevators, known as the body's natural mood lifters. This can lead to reductions in feelings of depression and anxiety

The psychological benefits of walking, such as enhanced mood and reduced symptoms of depression and anxiety, are linked to the increased release of endorphins and endocannabinoids—chemicals in the brain that act as natural painkillers and mood elevators. These substances can lead to what is often called the "runner's high," but similar effects can be achieved through brisk walking. This mood elevation is crucial for cognitive processes, as a positive mood has been shown to enhance creative thinking, problem-solving abilities, and memory recall.

The act of walking transcends mere physical activity; it is a potent modulator of brain function and mental health. Through mechanisms like enhanced cerebral blood flow, neurotrophic factor release, stress reduction, improved sleep quality, and the stimulation of neurogenesis, regular walking can significantly contribute to cognitive resilience and psychological well-being.

Walking is magic for the brain.

Expanding on chapter four when we first mentioned myo-kines and epigenetics, here's a little more information. When your muscles contract, they start a process that triggers the DNA, found in most of your cells, to make epigenetic changes. These temporary changes will result in the release of small proteins, also known as chemicals or hormones or genes or myokines from your muscle cells.

The myokines, (genes, hormones), make their way into the bloodstream. As they are carried through your body, some will make their way to the brain. Once in the brain they will affect different areas of the brain either alone or in concert with other myokines. Different areas of the brain control different functions.

The illustration below is not a map of the brain but is intended to show you how myokines get to the brain and the different brain functions affected by them. This is a highly complex process, and the drawing is intended to give you only a general understanding of the process.

The Exercise / Muscle Cell / Epigenetic / Myokine Pathway

Moderate exercise, such as walking, triggers a cascade of powerful chemicals (myokines) which will help your brain.

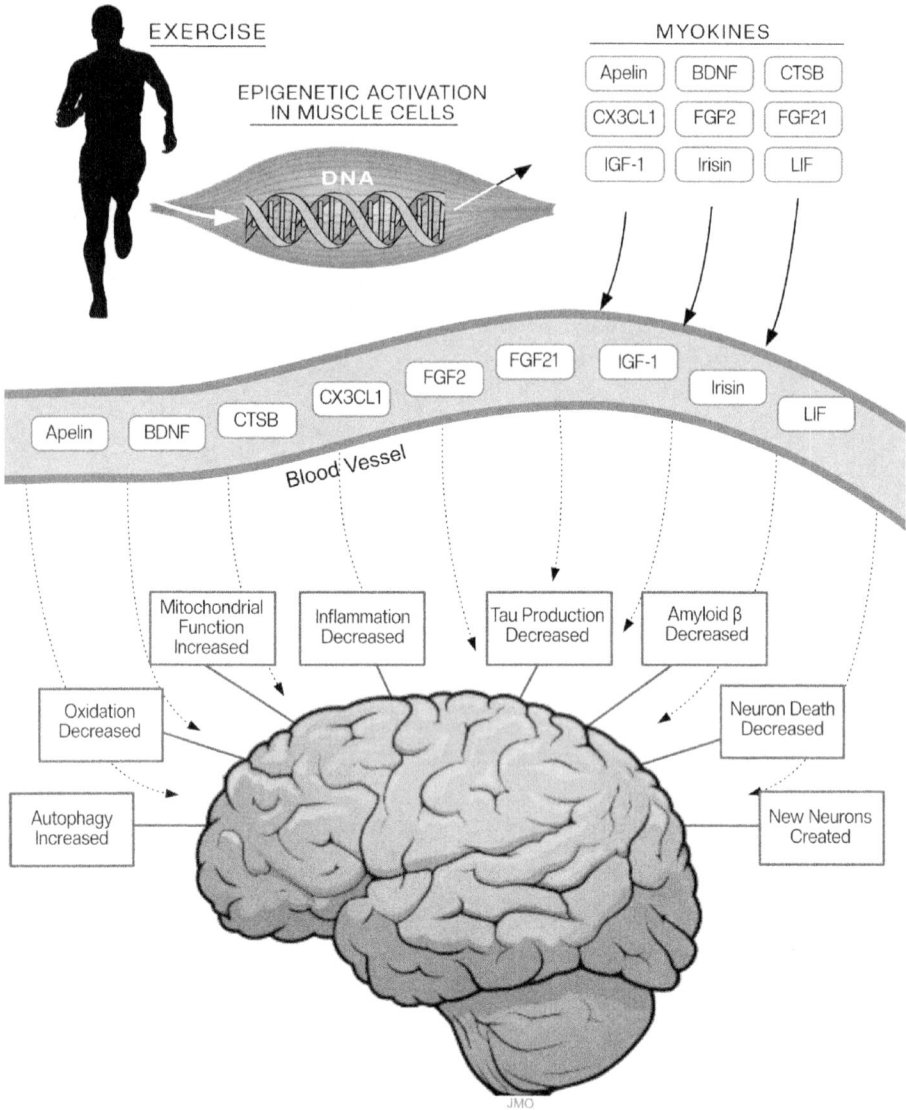

Remember, when everything is in balance–*that's homeostasis*–it works properly. That's the goal!

Cognitive fitness goes far beyond memory.
It embraces thinking, learning, recognition,
communication, and sound decision-making.
Cognitive fitness is the bedrock
of a rewarding, self-sufficient life.
Harvard University

Despite the robust. scientific evidence for the effectiveness of walking in the prevention and treatment of cognitive decline, we have no randomized clinical trials to prove that. And, chances are, we won't see any in the future because pharmaceutical companies can't sell walking.

I have a good friend who has Parkinson's Disease. He does boxing therapy, voice therapy, and ballet therapy. He walks a lot and stays in touch with old friends every week. Five years into the disease, he's doing great. If you don't know he has Parkinson's, you won't know.

Brisk walking and other forms of aerobic activity may not block or slow cognitive decline, but the evidence indicates it might. There is no doubt that walking and increased circulation will move you toward homeostasis, and *that* will move you toward better cognitive health.

A loss in cognitive function and a reduction in brain
volume is commonly observed in most
adults over the age of 65
Murman, 2015, Peters, 2006,

10 warning signs of dementia

1. Difficulty with everyday tasks. They may also find it hard to concentrate on tasks, take much longer to do them or have trouble finishing.

2. Repetition. Asking a question over and over or telling the same story about a recent event multiple times.

3. Communication problems. If a loved one has trouble joining or following a conversation, stops abruptly in the middle of a thought, or struggles to think of words or the name of objects.

4. Getting lost. People with dementia may have difficulty with visual and spatial abilities, such as getting lost while driving.

5. Personality changes. One who begins acting unusually anxious, confused, fearful or suspicious, becomes upset easil yor depressed.

6. Confusion about time and place. If someone forgets where they are or can't remember how they got there, that's a red flag. Another worrisome sign is disorientation about time — for example, routinely forgetting what day of the week it is.

7. Misplacing things. Someone with dementia may put things in unusual places and may have difficulty retracing their steps to find misplaced items, the Alzheimer's Association notes.

8. Troubling behavior. If your family member seems to have increasingly poor judgment when handling money or neglects grooming and cleanliness, pay attention.

9. Loss of interest, or apathy. Not feeling especially social from time to time is one thing, but a sudden and routine loss of interest in family, friends, work and social events is a warning sign of dementia.

10. Forgetting old memories. Memory loss that becomes more persistent is often one of the first signs of dementia.

10

Fantasy Walking and Treasure Hunting
Virtual Walking and Geocaching

When I first started walking every day, I started with relatively modest walks, but gradually increased to an average of about 25 miles per week. At this point, I thought, "If I walked 25 miles every week, I wonder how far that would be in a year's time." The answer — 1,300 miles — got me to wondering, "Where can I walk to that's 1,300 miles from Tulsa?" Hmmm, New York City is 1,343 miles according to Mr. Google, so I decided to celebrate my birthday that year by walking from Tulsa to New York. The previous year I celebrated my birthday by jumping out of an airplane at 10,000 feet, so, in comparison, this looked like a sensible decision.

I didn't *actually* walk from Tulsa to New York. It was a *fantasy* walk, a *virtual* walk. Every day I walk around my hometown (or whatever town I happen to be in) and then, every week or two, I plot my progress on a map I made for that purpose as shown below.

To help me feel more like I'm actually walking this trip, I used Google's Street View to virtually visit towns along the way. I learned a little about their history, saw their architecture and even snapped a few photos (screenshots of street views) of interesting buildings including churches, courthouses, theaters, houses and more. Every few weeks I would post some of this to

Facebook so my friends could see my progress and hold me accountable.

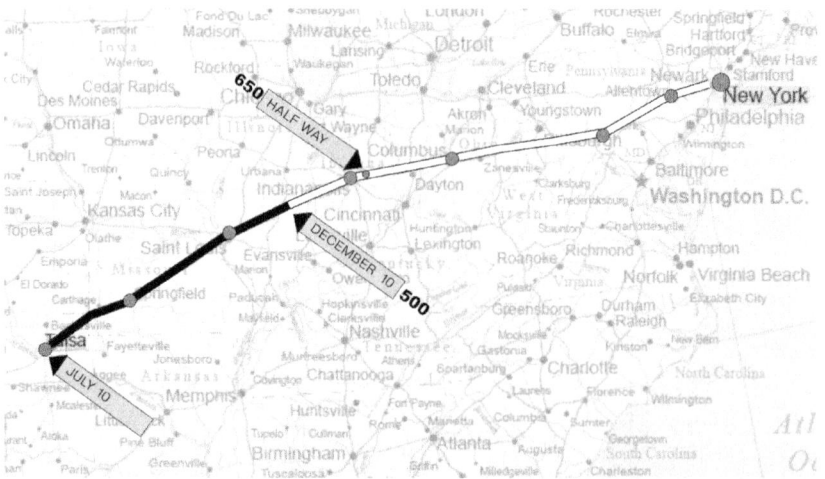

Why would you go to the trouble of inventing an imaginary walk? Couldn't you just set a goal of 25 miles per week and be done with it? Well sure, but where's the fun in that? This gives you a visible goal and it's a pretty BIG goal. It helps to motivate and focus your attention and it allows your friends to share in the experience. On the other hand, 25 miles per week as a goal can seem like drudgery!

As soon as I finished the New York trip, I immediately started on a Tulsa-to-Los Angeles trek. When I finished, I had virtually walked from New York to Los Angeles, a distance of 2,776 miles. While it is virtual, I *actually walked 2,776 miles!* At my age, at *any* age, I feel like that's a real accomplishment.

You don't need to limit your fantasy walks to such "pedestrian" choices (pun intended) as I have made. How about these walks —

London, England to Glasgow, Scotland – 367 miles

Paris, France to Rome, Italy – 1,461 miles

Addis Abada, Ethiopia to Djoubuti, Djoubuti – 470 miles

Baku, Azerbaijan to Tehran, Iran – 483 miles

The fun part of these trips will be virtually visiting towns along the way and learning about them. Baku and its flame-shaped buildings, for example, is absolutely amazing!

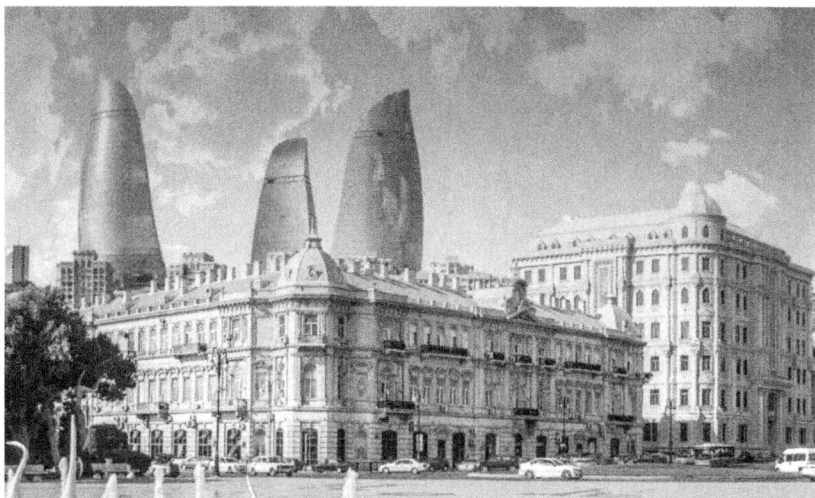

Now, let's talk about Geocaching

Geocaching is a lot like an Easter egg hunt, a treasure hunt, or an adult version of Hide and Seek or Pokémon GO. People all over the world have hidden geocaches for others to find using the GPS function on their smartphone.

There are more than 3 million cleverly hidden containers called geocaches hidden all over the world just waiting to be found. Geocaches come in all shapes and sizes—geocache creativity is endless—just look at the photos below! Some will be large reusable plastic or metal containers; others will be micro canisters hanging from a branch. Some will be as small as an acorn and *look exactly like an acorn*, while others mimic sticks, frogs, or industrial nuts and bolts (see photo). Make sure to read the size in your app to get on the right path. However, geocaches

A selection of geocashes including a camo-wrapped jar, a fake hollowed-out tree stump, a very realistic fake bolt-and-nut (hollow of course) which is usually attached by means of a magnet and the ever-popular ammo box. Standard Tupperware containers are also frequently used.

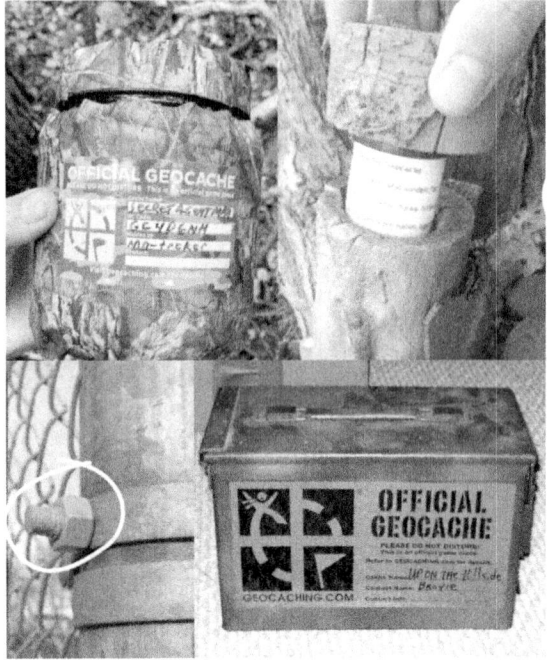

never require digging. The geocaches are all provided and placed by individuals in the global geocaching community. Some of these people are inventive, clever, accomplished artisans and some are just diabolical.

How you play Geocaching:

1. Open the app on your smartphone,

Or, alternately, you can simply log into their website, www.geocaching.com and start looking for geocaches on your phone. You can see from these two screenshots, there is a visual difference between using the app or the website. Once you select which one to use, then you…

2. Map your navigation to the geocache

Once you select a cache, go use the app to navigate to it. And don't forget to bring a pen so you can sign the logbook inside the geocache.

3. Look for the geocache

Once you make your way to the general location, use your phone to look at the recent activity and the hint for clues. Remember, geocaches come in all shapes and sizes!

4. Find and log the geocache

Once you find it, you'll need to open it and sign your username in the cache's logbook, then place the geocache back where you found it. Log your find in the app or on geocaching.com to see your find count increase!

What's inside a geocache depends on many things, especially the size of the geocache, but there should always be a log for you to sign. In larger caches, you can find trackables or items to trade. Trackables are meant to move from cache to cache. If you take something meant to be traded, make sure to leave something of equal or greater value!

Geocaching has many benefits. It's something you can do with your friends, children, or grandchildren. Chances are that they all could use some healthy, outside physical activities. Since it's primarily an outdoor recreational activity, it can be played in a safe, socially distant, COVID-19 acceptable way that adheres to your local laws and health guidance for outdoor activities.

Geocaching Website

Geocaching App

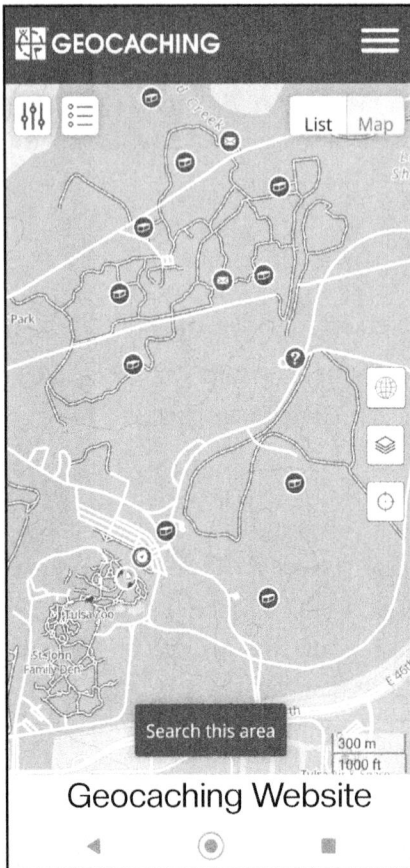

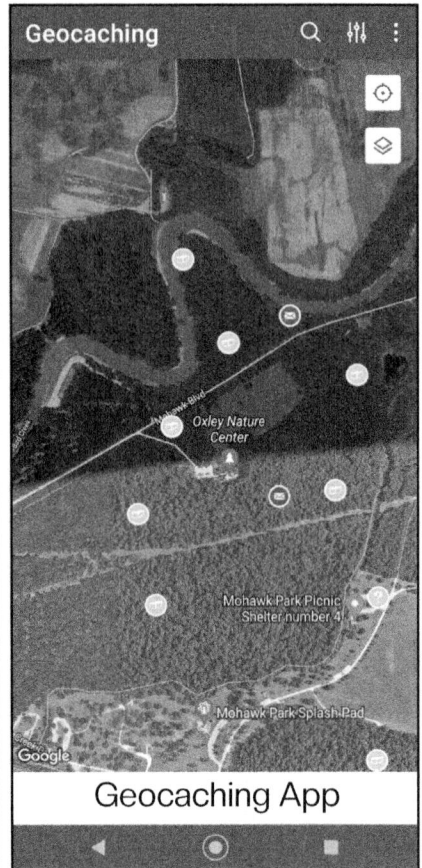

The screenshots shown above are of the Oxley Nature Center in Tulsa and show about a dozen caches in the area. Since the Oxley Center has more than ten miles of trails through woodlands, prairie and even marsh environments, you'll find ample opportunities to do some serious walking. Check to see the opportunities to be found in your nearby city, county, and state parks. In today's COVID-colored world, Geocaching is not only a welcomed social activity, but it can help improve mental fatigue from spending too much time indoors. Here are a couple of screenshots from the geocaching.com website that show the infinite opportunities the game presents.

Speaking of parks, they may have rules

State and national parks generally have varying policies regarding geocaching, which is a recreational activity involving the use of GPS devices to hide and seek containers, called "geocaches" or "caches," at specific locations marked by coordinates all over the world. While some parks embrace geocaching as a way to encourage outdoor exploration and engagement with nature, others may have restrictions or guidelines in place to manage its impact on the environment and visitor experience.

In parks where geocaching is allowed and even encouraged, participants may need to adhere to certain rules and guidelines to ensure the activity is conducted safely and responsibly. Common restrictions or guidelines related to geocaching in parks may include:

Permit Requirements: Some parks may require individuals or groups to obtain permits or permissions before placing geocaches within the park boundaries. This helps park authorities track the activity and ensure compliance with park regulations.

Environmental Protection: Geocachers are typically expected to follow Leave No Trace principles, which emphasize minimizing human impact on natural areas. This may include avoiding sensitive habitats, staying on designated trails, and properly disposing of any waste generated during the activity.

Safety Considerations: Parks may have specific safety guidelines related to geocaching, such as avoiding dangerous or off-limits areas, respecting wildlife, and being mindful of weather conditions and terrain difficulty.

Cache Placement and Size: Geocaches should be placed in accordance with park regulations, avoiding disturbance to natural features or cultural resources. Parks may also specify the maximum size and type of containers allowed for geocaches.

Notification and Monitoring: Geocachers may be required to notify park authorities of their intended geocache placements and provide details such as coordinates and descriptions. This allows park staff to monitor the activity and address any concerns or issues that may arise.

Walking is the closest thing we have to a Wonder Drug.

Thomas Frieden, MD, former director of the CDC

Overall, while geocaching can be a fun and rewarding activity for visitors to state and national parks, it's essential for participants to familiarize themselves with the specific policies and guidelines of each park they plan to visit. By respecting park regulations and practicing responsible geocaching, enthusiasts can enjoy the activity while minimizing its impact on the environment and ensuring a positive experience for themselves and others.

Running out of geocaches is not a likely possibility.

Geocaching started in May of 2000 when Dave Ulmer hid the first cache, known as the Original Stash, in Seattle. The activity quickly gained popularity, and caches began to appear not only in

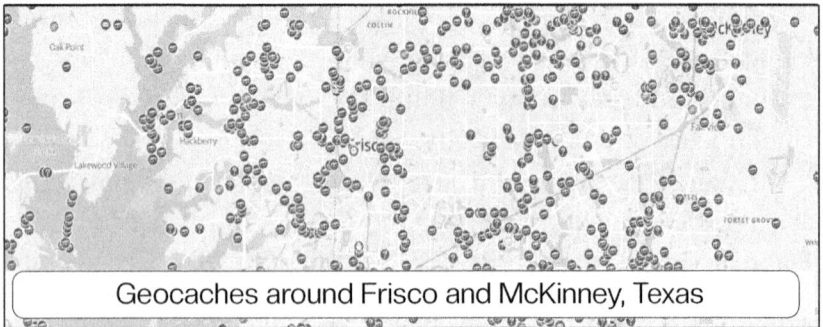

Geocaches around Frisco and McKinney, Texas

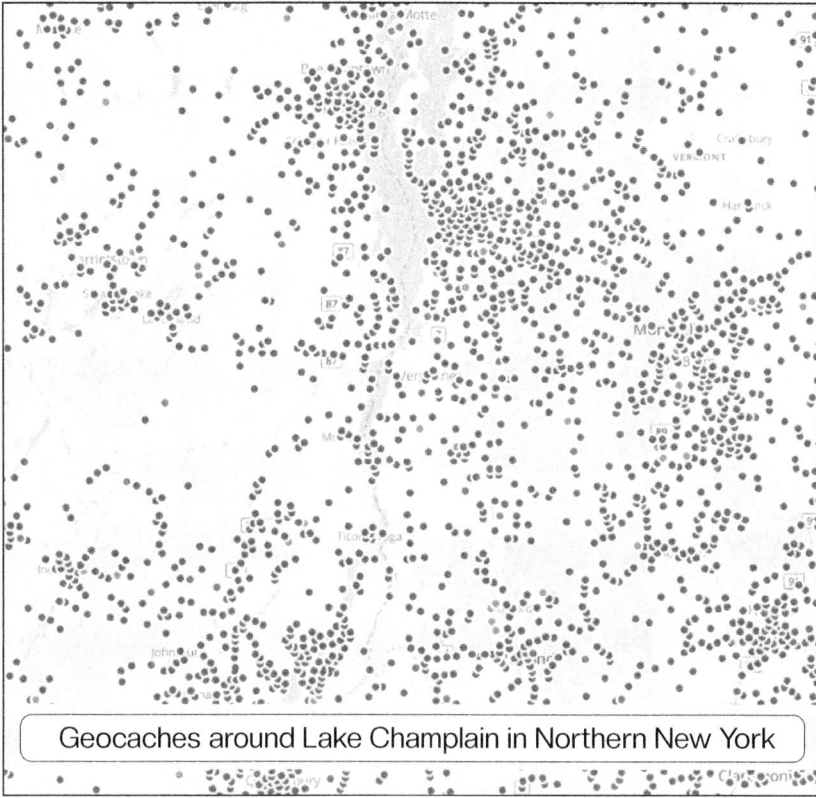

Geocaches around Lake Champlain in Northern New York

Washington but also throughout the world. Geocaching is now found in more than 200 countries but it is still headquartered in Seattle. Today, there are more than 24,000 caches in Washington and over three million more hidden all over the world. Wherever you live, it's highly likely that you will find a map of your area contains hundreds of caches.

Geocaching Merch!

You can find lots of merchandise for sale on the Geocaching website, (geocaching.com) and you can find even more on the Etsy site (1,600 items!), and hundreds more on Google and Amazon!

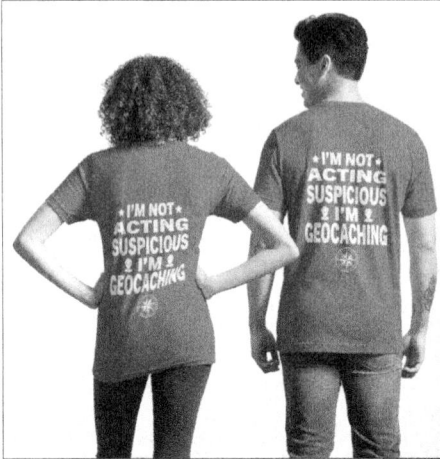

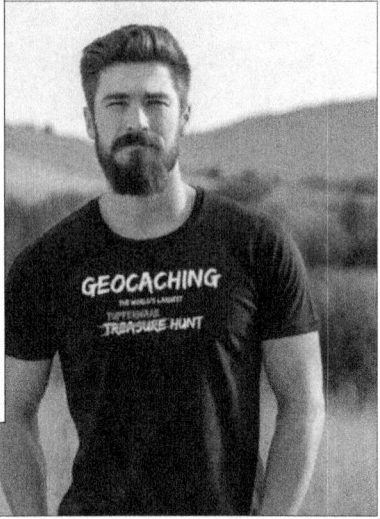

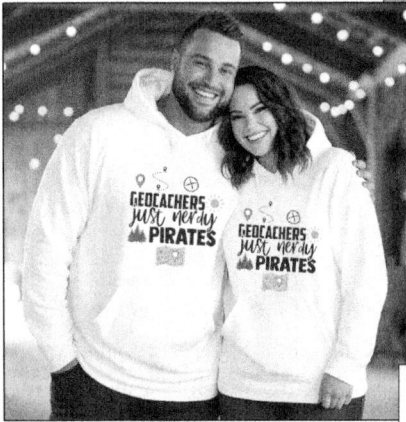

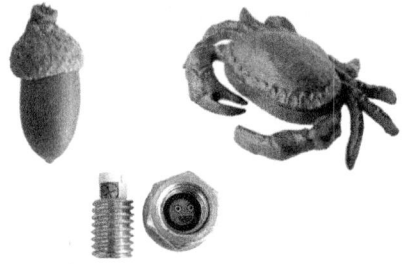

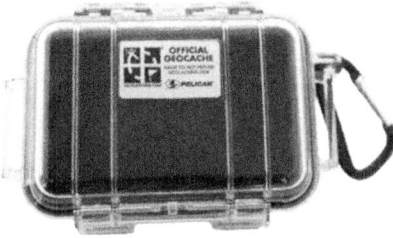

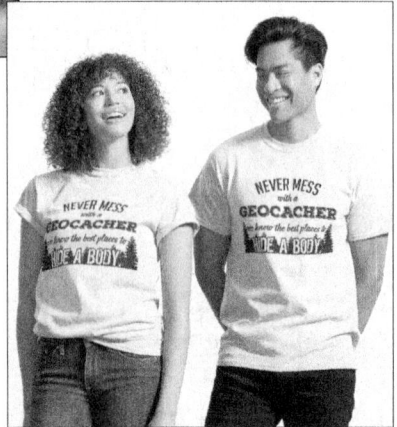

11

Irisin, the "Exercise Hormone"

In the pursuit of longevity and vitality, scientists have long sought to unravel the mysteries of aging and uncover strategies to promote healthspan—the period of life spent in good health. We've looked at some of their efforts, but there's a new kid in town shaking things up. The emerging star in this quest is called irisin. It's a myokine released by skeletal muscle during exercise, scientists are excited by its potential to enhance health and longevity through a myriad of cellular pathways.

*Note: this is a science-heavy chapter. It is not important that you understand the big medical words, just try to capture the overall picture of what **exercise+irisin** can do for you. The next chapter will be lighter, I promise!*

Bruce Spiegelman, a cellular biologist, and his colleagues at Dana-Farber Cancer Institute in Boston, discovered this new hormone in 2012 and named it "irisin," after Iris, the Greek messenger goddess. They foresaw the role of irisin as a "messenger." There has long been a feeling in the field that exercise 'talks to' various tissues in the body, but the question has been, *how*? His group's original discovery triggered an enormous amount of research into the role of irisin in the hope it can tell us exactly how. More than 2,000 studies released since 2012 show that the "exercise hormone" irisin has wide-ranging health benefits.

At the time of irisin's initial discovery, Spiegelman believed that it was an important first step in understanding the biological mechanisms that translate physical exercise into beneficial changes throughout the body in healthy people, and in preventing or treating disease.

Irisin has the ability to redirect your body's fat cells to burning energy instead of storing it by turning white fat cells (storage) to brown fat cells (energy-burning).

There is evidence that individuals with higher levels of irisin also have longer telomeres, the protective caps on the ends of their DNA, which is sometimes defined as being "biologically younger."

When irisin becomes elevated in your brain, through endurance exercise, it triggers the growth of new neurons (brain cells), in a process we have mentioned before, called neurogenesis which improves brain health and cognitive ability.

This great little hormone comes with two kinds of good news: first—it's a miracle-working hormone as we'll explain in depth later, that *you can make yourself*, and second—your body releases it in response to *moderate endurance aerobic activity*. Not the heavy-sweaty stuff.

And what is moderate endurance exercise? It includes any form of physical activity characterized by sustained, rhythmic movements that elevate heart rate and breathing for an extended period. It involves activities such as brisk walking, running, cycling, or swimming, which challenge the cardiovascular system. It also includes diverse activities such as dancing, gardening, golf, frisbee golf, pickleball, lawnmowing, vacuuming, and even hopscotch! Endurance exercise relies on aerobic metabolism to fuel muscle activity and sustain performance. Regular endurance exercise enhances cardiovascular health, builds stamina, and improves physical endurance. Its value to your body is probably underappreciated.

Metabolic Regulation

Irisin has garnered attention for its ability to regulate metabolism, particularly by promoting the conversion of white adipose tissue into metabolically active brown adipose tissue through a process known as browning or thermogenesis. This transformation enhances energy expenditure and contributes to the regulation of body weight and glucose homeostasis. Additionally, irisin has been shown to increase insulin sensitivity and glucose uptake in skeletal muscle, offering potential therapeutic implications for type 2 diabetes and metabolic syndrome.

Neuroprotective Effects

Irisin has emerged as a potential mediator of neuro-protection, exerting beneficial effects on brain health and cognitive function. Several studies have implicated irisin in promoting neurogenesis, the process by which new neurons are generated in the brain. It has been demonstrated that irisin can cross the blood-brain barrier and act directly on neural progenitor cells in the hippocampus, a brain region critical for learning and memory. Through its interaction with hippocampal cells, irisin stimulates the proliferation and differentiation of neural stem cells, leading to the generation of new neurons. This process, known as neurogenesis, plays a crucial role in maintaining cognitive function and has been implicated in the brain's ability to adapt to environmental stimuli and recover from injury.

"The act of walking transcends mere physical activity; it is a potent modulator of brain function and mental health."

A. Dietrich, W.F. McDaniel, 2004

Irisin has anti-inflammatory properties within the central nervous system, which may contribute to its brain-protective effects. Studies have demonstrated that irisin can suppress the activation of the immune cells of the brain, and inhibit the production of pro-inflammatory agents. By lowering brain inflammation, irisin helps preserve brain cell integrity and function, thereby protecting against neurodegenerative diseases such as Alzheimer's and Parkinson's disease. Additionally, irisin has been found to enhance synaptic plasticity, that's the ability of neurons to form and strengthen connections with one another, which is essential for learning and memory processes. Through its modulation of synaptic function, irisin may promote cognitive resilience and protect against age-related cognitive decline.

Emerging evidence suggests that irisin may play a role in controlling brain-derived neurotrophic factor (BDNF) signaling, a key pathway involved in brain cell survival, growth, and plasticity. Irisin has been shown to increase the expression of BDNF and its receptor in the brain, thereby promoting brain cell survival and synaptic plasticity. By enhancing BDNF signaling, irisin supports the maintenance of healthy brain function and protects against neurodegenerative disorders. Overall, the brain-protective effects of irisin highlight its potential as a therapeutic agent for the prevention and treatment of cognitive decline and neurodegenerative diseases.

Cardiovascular Health

Irisin has emerged as a key regulator of cardiovascular health. Studies have shown that irisin exerts beneficial effects on the cardiovascular system through various mechanisms. One of its primary roles is the promotion of endothelial function, which is essential for maintaining the health and integrity of blood vessels. Irisin has been found to enhance endothelial cell function by increasing the production of nitric oxide (NO), a potent vasodilator that relaxes blood vessels, thereby improving blood flow and reducing vascular resistance. Additionally, irisin has been shown to inhibit endothelial cell apoptosis and inflammation, further contributing to vascular health.

Furthermore, irisin has been implicated in the regulation of fat metabolism and the prevention of atherosclerosis, a major risk factor for cardiovascular disease. Studies have demonstrated that irisin can modulate lipid metabolism by promoting the expression of genes involved in fatty acid oxidation and inhibiting lipid accumulation in vascular cells. This anti-atherogenic effect of irisin is attributed to its ability to activate AMPK, a key regulator of cellular energy metabolism, and inhibit the expression of pro-inflammatory cytokines and adhesion molecules in vascular endothelial cells.

Moreover, irisin has been shown to possess anti-hypertensive properties, which may contribute to its overall cardioprotective effects. Animal studies have revealed that irisin administration can reduce blood pressure in hypertensive models by enhancing endothelium-dependent vasodilation and suppressing sympathetic nervous system activity. These findings suggest that irisin plays a crucial role in maintaining cardiovascular homeostasis and protecting against the development of cardiovascular diseases.

Activation of SIRT1

Irisin has been found to activate the SIRT1 pathway, a key regulator of cellular metabolism and longevity. SIRT1, a member of the sirtuin family of proteins, plays a central role in various physiological processes, including energy metabolism, DNA repair, and stress response. Activation of SIRT1 by irisin promotes mitochondrial biogenesis and enhances oxidative metabolism in skeletal muscle cells, leading to improved energy production and endurance capacity. Additionally, SIRT1 activation by irisin has been linked to enhanced insulin sensitivity and glucose homeostasis, which may contribute to its beneficial effects on metabolic health.

Additionally, irisin-induced activation of SIRT1 has been implicated in the regulation of cellular senescence and aging-related pathways. Studies have demonstrated that irisin *can attenuate cellular senescence* by inhibiting the expression of senescence-associated markers and promoting cell survival and proliferation. This anti-aging effect of irisin is mediated, at least in part, through its ability to activate SIRT1, which in turn deacetylates and activates downstream targets involved in cellular stress resistance and longevity. By modulating SIRT1 activity, irisin may help counteract age-related decline in tissue function and promote healthy aging.

Emerging evidence suggests that irisin-mediated activation

of SIRT1 may confer neuroprotective effects and enhance cognitive function. SIRT1 has been implicated in various neuroprotective pathways, including synaptic plasticity, mitochondrial function, and antioxidant defense. Activation of SIRT1 by irisin in the brain has been shown to promote neuronal survival, enhance synaptic plasticity, and improve cognitive performance in animal models of neurodegenerative diseases. These findings suggest that irisin-SIRT1 signaling axis may represent a promising target for the development of novel therapeutic interventions for age-related neurodegenerative disorders. *11.9*

Activation of AMPK- Metabolic Flexibility and Stress Resistance

Irisin has garnered significant attention for its role in modulating cellular energy metabolism and cardiovascular health. One of its key mechanisms of action involves the activation of AMP-activated protein kinase (AMPK), a master regulator of cellular energy homeostasis. Upon secretion, irisin can stimulate AMPK signaling pathways in various tissues, including the heart and blood vessels. Activation of AMPK by irisin leads to a cascade of downstream effects that promote energy production, glucose uptake, and lipid metabolism, ultimately contributing to improved cardiovascular function.

Studies have demonstrated that irisin-mediated activation of AMPK exerts protective effects on the cardiovascular system by enhancing endothelial function and reducing vascular inflammation. AMPK activation by irisin has been shown to promote endothelial nitric oxide synthase (eNOS) activity, leading to increased nitric oxide (NO) production and vasodilation. Additionally, irisin-induced AMPK activation can inhibit the expression of pro-inflammatory cytokines and adhesion molecules in endothelial cells, thereby attenuating endothelial dysfunction and vascular inflammation. Irisin-AMPK signaling helps maintain vascular health and prevent the development of cardiovascular diseases.

Furthermore, irisin-induced activation of AMPK has been implicated in the regulation of cardiac energy metabolism and contractile function. Studies in animal models have demonstrated that irisin administration can improve cardiac mitochondrial function, increase myocardial (heart muscle) glucose uptake, and enhance cardiac contractility through AMPK-dependent mechanisms. These cardioprotective effects of irisin may have implications for the prevention and treatment of heart failure and other cardiovascular conditions. Overall, the irisin-AMPK axis represents a promising therapeutic target for modulating cardiovascular health and combating metabolic disorders.

Through AMPK activation, irisin enhances glucose uptake, fatty acid oxidation, and mitochondrial biogenesis, thereby improving metabolic flexibility and mitigating age-related metabolic dysfunction.

Induction of Autophagy: Cleaning Up Cellular Junk for Longevity

Irisin has garnered attention for its role in inducing autophagy, (aw-TOFF-a-gee) a cellular process crucial for maintaining cellular homeostasis and promoting longevity. Autophagy, often referred to as cellular self-cleansing, or "taking out the trash" involves the degradation and recycling of damaged or dysfunctional cellular components to generate energy and maintain cellular function. Studies have demonstrated that irisin can stimulate autophagy in various cell types, including muscle cells, neurons, and adipocytes (fat cells). By enhancing autophagic activity, irisin helps to remove accumulated cellular debris, mitigate oxidative stress, and promote cellular repair and regeneration.

The induction of autophagy by irisin has been linked to a myriad of health benefits, including improved metabolic health, enhanced mitochondrial function, and protection against age-related diseases. Autophagy plays a critical role in regulating energy metabolism by promoting the breakdown of cellular components to generate nutrients and energy during periods of nutrient deprivation or metabolic stress. Irisin-mediated activation of autophagy has been shown to enhance lipid metabolism and insulin sensitivity, thereby improving metabolic health and reducing the risk of obesity and type 2 diabetes. Additionally, autophagy is essential for maintaining mitochondrial integrity and function, as dysfunctional mitochondria are targeted for degradation through the autophagic process. By promoting mitochondrial turnover and biogenesis, irisin-induced autophagy helps to maintain cellular energy production and prevent the accumulation of damaged mitochondria, thereby enhancing overall metabolic health and longevity.

Furthermore, emerging evidence suggests that irisin-induced autophagy may have neuroprotective effects and promote brain health. Autophagy plays a crucial role in removing misfolded proteins and damaged organelles from neurons, thereby preventing the accumulation of toxic aggregates and preserving neuronal function. Irisin-mediated activation of autophagy has been shown to protect against neurodegenerative diseases such as Alzheimer's and Parkinson's disease by clearing protein aggregates and promoting neuronal survival. Moreover, autophagy is essential for synaptic plasticity and neuronal adaptation, processes that are critical for learning and memory. The irisin-enhanced autophagic activity in the brain, is another way that irisin promotes cognitive function and protects against age-related cognitive decline.

Irisin activation of telomerase: safeguarding chromosomes and aiding longevity

Irisin is a key regulator of telomerase activity, an enzyme essential for maintaining chromosome integrity and promoting longevity. Telomerase (tel-OH-mer-aze, or tel-AH-mer-aze) plays a crucial role in preserving telomere (TEE-lo-mere) length, the protective caps at the ends of chromosomes that shorten with each cell division and serve as markers of cellular aging. Studies have demonstrated that irisin can increase telomerase expression and activity in various cell types, including muscle cells, neurons, and immune cells. By enhancing telomerase activity, irisin helps to prevent telomere shortening, *delay cellular senescence*, and promote cellular longevity.

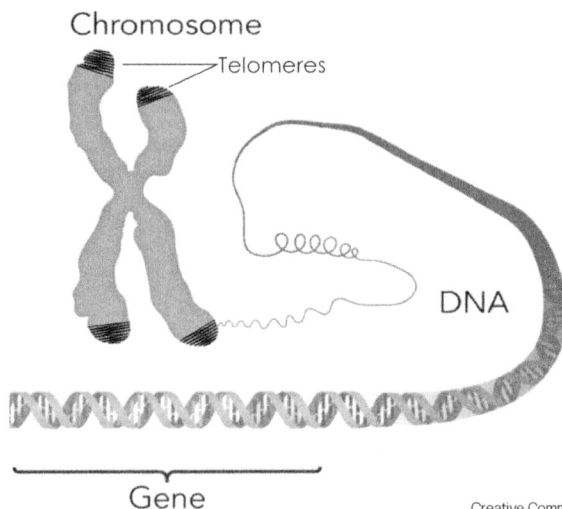

Chromosome
Telomeres
DNA
Gene

The activation of telomerase by irisin has profound implications for overall health and longevity, as telomere length is closely associated with aging and age-related diseases. Shortened telomeres have been linked to an increased risk of age-related diseases, including cardiovascular disease, diabetes, and cancer, as well as accelerated aging and premature mortality. By preserving telomere length and protecting against telomere erosion, irisin-induced activation of telomerase may help to delay the onset of age-related diseases and extend healthy lifespan. Moreover, telomerase activation has been shown to enhance cellular stress resistance, improve DNA repair capacity, and promote tissue regeneration, all of which contribute to improved healthspan and longevity.

Another amazing fact:

If you look at the diagram on the previous page of a chromosome, you will noticed that a chromosome is a DNA that has been twisted, wound, scrunched, and woven into an X shape. On each end of the X there are little booties. Scientists call them telomeres.

The DNA in each human cell has to be copied every time a cell divides—that's mitosis, remember?—which occurs nearly 300 billion times each day.* Each of these new cells contains 46 chromosomes. Do the math: 300 billion x 46 = about 14 trillion new DNA *every day.* If errors occur in DNA replication, cells can become abnormal and cause disease. —

*Scientific American, April 2021.

Irisin-mediated activation of telomerase is involved in the regulation of immune function and inflammation, processes that play crucial roles in aging and age-related diseases. Telomerase activity is essential for maintaining immune cell function and preventing immune senescence, which can lead to impaired immune responses and increased susceptibility to infections and chronic diseases. Studies have shown that irisin can enhance telomerase activity in immune cells, such as T cells and macrophages, thereby promoting immune cell longevity and function. By bolstering immune cell integrity and function, irisin helps to mitigate age-related immune dysfunction and inflammation, contributing to overall health and longevity.

A little more info about telomeres: they are structures located at the ends of chromosomes, consisting of repetitive DNA sequences and associated proteins. Their primary function is to protect the chromosome during cell division by preventing them from deteriorating or fusing with neighboring chromosomes. Telomeres also play a crucial role in cellular aging and lifespan regulation. With each cell division, telomeres gradually shorten, eventually reaching a critically short length. Shortened telomeres have been linked to age-related diseases and overall mortality risk, making them a key marker of biological aging. It is believed that a person can help maintaining telomere length through various lifestyle factors, such as healthy diet, regular exercise, and, of course, irisin.

All these benefits from one little myokine — and there are more than 600 myokines?

Yes, isn't it amazing? You may have noticed there are a lot of overlapping and redundant interactions between all these chemicals. While your doctor may give you one, two or three drugs, your body's "inner pharmacy" can give you *dozens* with perfect dosages and physiological combinations to match your body's needs.

That's a great return on a little physical activity.

12

Rucking: Good to the Bone

Rucking is a new version of an old form of exercise. It involves walking or hiking with a weighted backpack where the extra weight turns a normal walk into an amplified form of exercise.

Rucking (also known as ruck marching) evolved from military training in the seventh century B.C., and the name comes from rucksack, a durable backpack meant for carrying heavy loads. Ruck comes from *ruken,* the German word for back. The ability to march long distances carrying a load of equipment has historically been central to most military units and is still a part of military training today.

In the armed forces, ruck marches involve carrying a load of standard military issue gear over a given distance. In basic training, Army rangers are required to carry a 35-pound rucksack 12 miles in less than three hours (15 minutes per mile).

Civilian backpacks used for rucking tend to be lighter with more comfortable straps. Military backpacks usually have metal or plastic frames.

When rucking, you'll experience less pounding on the knees than when running, making rucking a good choice for low-impact exercise. The added weight also requires more force and stamina, too.

Rucking improves strength, endurance, and general fitness. For example, a 2019 study found participants had lower ratings of perceived exertion after a 10-week load carrying program, while their muscle power and oxygen intake also improved.

Rucking has also been shown to improve muscle power in older people. This research implies rucking could offer an effective training program for preventing sarcopenia (muscle wasting) as well as degenerative bone conditions (osteopenia and osteoporosis) that can lead to falls and injuries in senior populations.

Walking with weight also increases the number of calories you burn compared to your normal walk. The added weight means you have more mass to move which increases the amount of energy needed to move compared to walking without the weight.

If you are new to exercising or haven't hiked much, then it is best to start slowly. Start with a walk of about two miles. Load your backpack with about 10% of your body weight. For instance, if you weigh 170 pounds, you should load your pack with 17 pounds.

For weight, you can use dumbbells, kettlebells, sandbags, bricks, rocks, or bottles of water. I use bricks which weigh about 4.5 pounds each. Four of them are close to 10% of my body weight. For the best results, secure the weight so that it doesn't move or bounce around. If you think you'll be rucking often, you may want to consider investing in a backpack and weights that are meant specifically for this purpose. Here's an example of how a backpack frame might look.

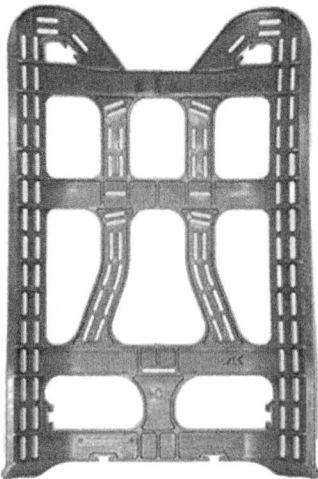

Companies such as Goruck, make rucksacks and weight plates that are ergonomically designed specifically for even distribution of weight. The Empack by Evolved Motion comes with reservoirs you can fill with water or sand to create the weight you'd like, and you can even change it while hiking.

When your fitness begins to improve, you can slowly increase the amount of weight you carry, the speed you're walking, or the distance you are rucking. To avoid the possibility of overtraining, increase only one of these at a time. If your goal is to increase strength, focus on increasing the load weight. If, on the other hand, your goal is to increase endurance, add distance to your ruck.

Rucking can burn more calories than running.

According to US Army figures, a 180-pound person rucking at a pace of 15 minutes per mile (four miles per hour) will burn the following calories:

Pack weight:	35 pounds	50 pounds	70 pounds
Ruck 3.7 miles	680 calories	735 calories	820 calories
Ruck 8 miles	1360 calories	1475 calories	1635 calories
Ruck 12 miles	2040 calories	2210 calories	2455 calories

Let's compare rucking to running: A 180-pound person running at a pace of 6 miles per hour (equal to 10 minutes per mile) *without* weight will burn roughly 840 calories per hour. That equals about 140 calories per mile.

To cover the same ground as listed in the chart above, a 180-pound person running at the pace of 6 miles per hour with a 70-pound backpack would burn 518 calories over 3.7 miles, 1120 calories over 8 miles, and 1680 calories over 12 miles. That's 46% more calories burned through rucking compared to running.

While your calorie burn has some variables, rucking obviously can burn more calories than running.

> Numerous studies have shown that weight-bearing exercise can help to slow bone loss, and several show it can even build bone. Activities that put stress on bones stimulate extra deposits of calcium and nudge bone-forming cells into action. The tugging and pushing on bone that occur during strength and power training provide the stress. The result is stronger, denser bones.
>
> —Harvard Health Website

The Benefits of Rucking

Rucking may be one of your best choices for preventing bone deterioration or restoring your bone strength. There are two key aspects an activity must have for protecting or restoring bones: first, it must be a *weight-bearing* exercise, which activates a process known as bone remodeling. Weight-bearing in this context mainly means you are working against gravity by walking, jogging, stair climbing, dancing, or sports such as pickleball or tennis; secondly, it is best if the exercise has *impact*, such as happens when your feet strike the ground when walking. The addition of weight in rucking serves as a *multiplier of both weight-bearing and impact.*

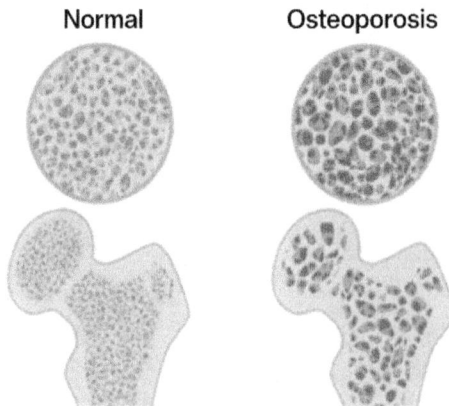

Normal   **Osteoporosis**

The importance of bone health becomes more apparent as we age. This is when we encounter bone deterioration in the form of *osteopenia* and *osteoporosis,* a weakening of the bones. This can become a significant concern, especially in postmenopausal women.

Bone Deteriorates with Age:

Decreased Calcium Absorption: Aging can lead to decreased calcium absorption in the gut, which is essential for bone health. This can further exacerbate bone density loss.

Changes in Bone Microstructure: Aging affects the microarchitecture of bones. The trabecular bone (the spongy part inside bones) becomes less dense, reducing bone strength and making fractures more likely.

Alterations in Bone Remodeling: The balance between bone resorption (breakdown) and bone formation becomes disrupted with age. Osteoclasts, responsible for breaking down old bone, may become more active while osteoblasts, responsible for building new bone, may become less efficient.

Risk Factors: In addition to aging, several factors increase the risk of osteoporosis, including family history, low body weight, smoking, excessive alcohol consumption, and certain medications (e.g., corticosteroids).

Fracture Risk: Osteoporosis can lead to debilitating fractures, particularly in the spine (vertebral fractures), hip, and wrist. These fractures can result from minor falls or even normal daily activities and can have severe consequences for an individual's quality of life.

Controlling Bone Deterioration:

Exercise is a crucial component of maintaining bone health, especially as you age. Here's how it helps:

Weight-bearing exercises, such as walking, running, dancing, rucking and, to a lesser degree, weight training, put stress on your bones. This stress stimulates bone cells (osteoblasts) to *build new bone* and strengthens existing bone. Regular weight-bearing exercise can help *maintain bone density* and can even increase it.

Weight-bearing exercises also influence the structure of bones. They help *align the collagen fibers* within bones in a way that enhances their strength and resistance to stress. This improved bone architecture reduces the risk of fractures and increases overall bone strength.

Weight-bearing exercise promotes *better mineralization* of bones, especially the deposition of calcium and other minerals. This mineralization process strengthens the bone matrix, making it more durable.

Weight-bearing exercise stimulates the *release of hormones* such as growth hormone and insulin-like growth factor (IGF-1). These hormones play crucial roles in bone health by promoting bone growth and remodeling.

Exercise is the most efficient intervention to improve muscle function and whole-body metabolism.

Egan, Zierath, 2013,

The mechanical stress generated through rucking and other activities during weight-bearing exercises triggers *bone adaptation*. Bones respond to this stress by becoming *denser* and *stronger* in areas that are subjected to the most load.

Exercise programs that include balance and coordination training can *reduce the risk of falls and fractures* in older adults.

These activities, such as Tai Chi, yoga, and rucking can improve your stability and help prevent accidents.

Building and maintaining muscle strength through rucking and weight training can indirectly benefit bone health. Strong muscles provide better support to your bones and reduce the risk of falling, which can lead to fractures. (Every year, nearly one third of Americans over the age of 65 experience a fall, and 88 people die from falls per day!)

While aerobic activities like swimming or cycling don't directly impact bone density because they are *not weight-bearing*, they contribute to overall health and fitness, which can enhance your ability to engage in weight-bearing exercises and maintain an active lifestyle. Rucking, of course, combines both weight-bearing and aerobic benefits.

> "I've also become semiobsessed with an activity
> called rucking, which basically means hiking
> or walking at a fast pace with a loaded pack
> on your back, three or four days a week"
> Peter Attia, MD, *Outlive*

Rucking over time will stimulate your bones to adapt to the increased load, stress, and impact, leading to several mechanisms that contribute to stronger bones. Rucking is now looking pretty good for getting your bones into shape, right?

But wait, there's more! Rucking is a low-impact activity, meaning it puts less stress on your joints compared to high-impact activities such as running or jumping. This makes it a suitable option for individuals who may have joint issues or are looking for a lower-impact way to strengthen their bones.

Carrying a backpack during rucking benefits multiple muscle groups, including those in your legs, core, and upper body. This muscle engagement not only helps strengthen muscles but can also provide better support for your bones.

You can adjust the weight of your backpack to control the intensity of your rucking workouts. Gradually increasing the load as you progress can help your bones adapt to greater stress and become stronger over time.

Rucking has practical applications, as it simulates carrying a load, which is a common activity in daily life or during outdoor adventures like hiking or camping. Building bone strength through rucking can improve your ability to engage in other activities.

To incorporate rucking into an overall plan for bone strength, consider the following tips:

Start Slowly: If you're new to rucking, begin with a lighter load and shorter distances to allow your body to adapt gradually. As you become more comfortable, you can increase the weight and duration of your rucking sessions.

Maintain Proper Form: Pay attention to your posture and form while rucking. Keep your back straight, shoulders relaxed, and distribute the weight evenly in your backpack to prevent strain or injury.

Include Variety: Combine rucking with other weight-bearing exercises like walking, hiking, pickleball, tennis, bowling, or strength training to create a well-rounded bone-strengthening routine.

Consult a Professional: If you have any underlying medical conditions or concerns about your bone health, it's advisable to consult with a healthcare provider or fitness professional to ensure your exercise plan aligns with your specific needs.

Stay Consistent: Consistency is key to reaping the benefits of rucking for bone strength. Aim to incorporate it into your weekly exercise routine to see long-term improvements in bone density and overall bone health.

Remember that bone health is influenced by many diverse factors, including diet, genetics, and overall lifestyle. Combining rucking with a balanced diet rich in calcium and vitamin D, as well as other weight-bearing exercises and activities, can contribute to strong and healthy bones as you age.

Before choosing an activity, it is important to consider your risk of falling. Your doctor, physical therapist, or athletic trainer can help you plan your exercise program. People with severe osteoporosis should be careful when rucking to avoid excessive spine compression.

13

The BrainHealth Project

Throughout history, it had been assumed that humans are born with all the brain cells they will ever have. In 1998, however, Fred Gage and Peter Eriksson discovered that the human brain produces new nerve cells in adulthood — the process we call neurogenesis.

Neurons are born as blank-slate stem cells and they go through a development process where they must find something to do in order to survive — and most of them don't. It takes about four weeks for a newborn cell to plug into a neural network and the old saying, "use 'em or lose 'em" is absolutely true for neurons.

Exercise gives birth to neurons, but "in order for a cell to fire and integrate, it has to fire its axon," Gage says, which means it has to carry a new message with new information. It is only through stimulation and environmental enrichment that those new cells survive. In other words, the survival of those new brain cells is all up to you. It's time to exercise your brain!

You can accomplish this in several ways. You can read books, work crosswords, play Sudoku, join a Tai Chi course, meet new people, learn a new language or more. There are several web sites offering mind-improving games such as Brain HQ, Lumosity, and the AARP's Staying Sharp program. Or, you could opt for a personal trainer for your brain, well, sort of.

The Center for BrainHealth® – part of The University of Texas at Dallas – is a nonprofit research institute redefining how people understand and address the brain's health and performance. Their team conducts leading-edge research and creates science-backed programs that empower people to be more proactive about their own brain health. The Center has spent three decades and millions of dollars developing a program, called the **BrainHealth Project.** It's an open-access, ongoing study, similar to "a personal trainer for your brain" and, best of all, it's free! They currently have more than 25,000 people enrolled with a target of 100,000, and the goal of tracking people for ten years to build a database of how people respond to various methods designed to improve their brains.

Our brains start to decline as early as our 20's or 30's; cognitive neuroscience research, however, has shown us that decline is not inevitable if we practice brain-healthy strategies.

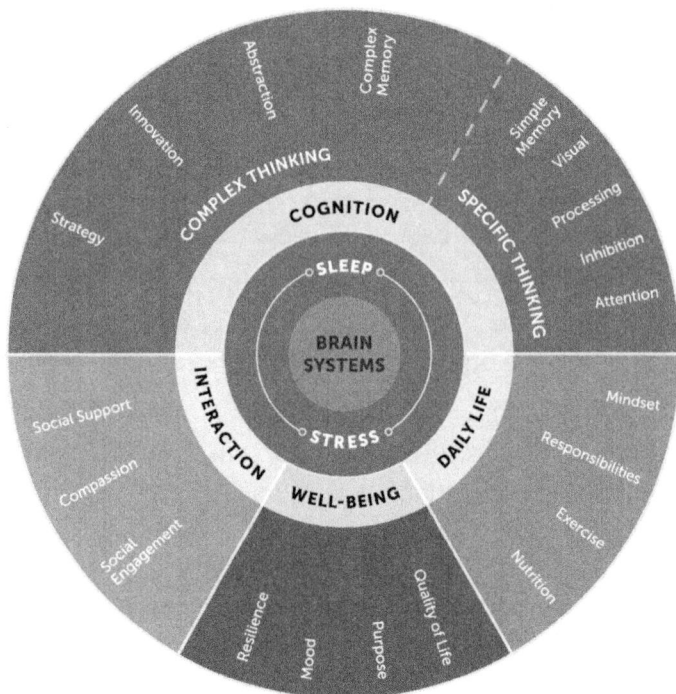

Early results from The BrainHealth Project, show that 80% of participants experience a meaningful improvement in their BrainHealth Index – a proprietary tool, the first holistic, science-backed measure to track improvement in brain health. Traditional thinking about brain health is rooted in the medical model, focusing on disease, disorder and deficits. BrainHealth researchers have determined that interventions shown to help populations with specific deficits also helped people with different deficits.

I never considered that having a brain health coach could improve mental performance, just as my yoga instructor and golf coach help me improve in those areas ... I feel like my brain health and overall well-being are moving in the right direction, and that feels good at any age.
Ben, a Brain Health Project participant.

Eventually, their research led to the discovery that these interventions can even help healthy people strengthen their brain health — that better brain health helps people thrive within the context of their personal life. The project is reframing the definition of brain health: it's about making the most of your capacity to thrive in life.

BrainHealth Index: A 21st Century Metric

The concept of IQ might have been useful 100 years ago when it was developed, when repetitive, assembly-line work was the norm and the ability to remember a lot of information was prized.

But this concept is limiting – today, complex skills such as adaptability, innovation, meaningful social connection, and deriving meaning from data are the strongest drivers of success, not to mention our ability to use computers and phones to store and retrieve almost infinite amounts of data.

So what is the "IQ test" for the 21st century?

BrainHealth researchers developed the BrainHealth Index: the world's first multifaceted performance metric for the integrated, complex brain functions that are directed by the brain's frontal networks.

Exercise is the single most powerful tool
you have to optimize your brain function
John J. Ratey, MD, *Spark*

Decline Is Not Inevitable

At the Center for BrainHealth, cognitive neuroscientists have teamed up with clinicians to translate scientific findings into real-world applications.

Common thinking once held that after our mid-20s, the only brain change possible was decline. In the late 1990s science began to reveal the power of neuroplasticity, and researchers started exploring the extent to which the brain can grow stronger, adapt and work better throughout our lifespan.

Strategic Memory Advanced Reasoning Tactics, or SMART™, teaches strategies to calibrate mental energy, reinforce strategic thinking and ignite innovation.

Brain Health Builds on Multiple Domains

The components of brain health include cognition, daily life, well-being and interaction with others.

It is still common to envision a healthy brain as a set of pillars – all equally important and seeming to function independently. However, research demonstrates that the multiple components of the brain's health are tightly integrated, and that cognitive fitness creates change across all the components. Because cognition is the way we perceive and engage with the world, this component undergirds the others.

Hands down, the most important intervention
we have for aging, is exercise.
Nir Barzilai, *Age Later*

The BrainHealth team conducts research and creates science-backed programs that help people to be more proactive about their own brain health. The fact that human longevity has increased more than 50% in the last century means that our bodies often outlast our brains. According to the American Heart Association, in 2020, fifty-four million people worldwide had Alzheimer's disease or other dementias—a 144-percent increase in the last thirty years.

"With increasing longevity and the aging of the Baby Boom generation, *cognitive impairment is projected to increase significantly over the next few decades,"* says Jennifer Manly, PhD, professor of neuropsychology at the Taub Institute for Research on Alzheimer's Disease and the Aging Brain at Columbia University, "affecting individuals, families, and programs that provide care and services for people with dementia," The economic impact of dementia, including unpaid family caregiving, is estimated to be $257 billion per year in the United States

Many research studies have shown that cognitive decline is *largely preventable*. The Brain Health Project hopes to prove that most of us can, by adopting healthier brain habits, preserve, extend, and even improve our cognitive function.

Their website describes the BrainHealth Project as a scientific study to measure and track one's own brain fitness. Nearly 80% of participants in an early trial experienced signs of improved cognitive performance, with many also noting reductions in stress and anxiety.

Their easy-to-use online platform gives you access to:

A unique, science-backed assessment of your brain's fitness level that they call the BrainHealth Index, that will provide you a snapshot of your brain's health and performance, allowing you (and them) to track any changes and improvements over time.

Day by day (or longer, it's self-paced), you will progress through interactive, self-paced brain training using what they call Strategic Memory Advanced Reasoning Tactics (SMART)™ Brain Training and other modules.

Quarterly face-to-face virtual coaching sessions via Zoom to set personal goals, and then start building brain-healthy habits using their online training on topics such as sleep, stress management and social relationships.

SMART™ Brain Training is the proprietary methodology developed and tested by the Center for BrainHealth researchers and other teams over three decades. It teaches techniques that prime the brain, calibrate mental energy, reinforce strategic thinking, and ignite innovation. This methodology provides the building blocks of their brain training programs for individual and

When you enroll in the brain health program, you might be surprised to learn that there is an opportunity for engagement every day, and they're not bashful about encouraging you to keep working on your training. They send reminders both as text messages and as emails. They have topics such as Strategic Attention,

Integrated Reasoning, Innovation, and application of SMART Strategies. Each session has a short video introduction explaining the purpose of that session, followed by a variety of brain tasks. Each group of tasks takes five to ten minutes and you're expected to do one a day.

You'll have a one-on-one Zoom coaching session every six months. My first Zoom coaching session was pretty minimal. Basically, she asked if I had any questions. I asked if a particular test on which I did poorly, would be something I would encounter again. She assured me that I would.

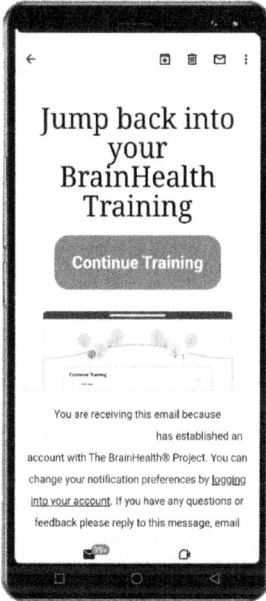

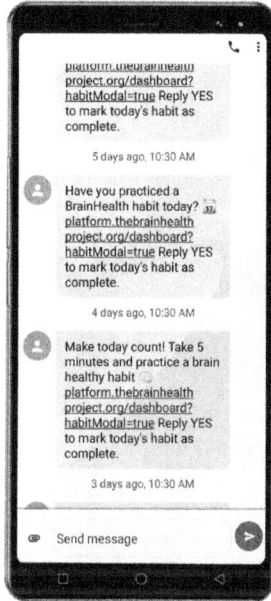

At my next coaching meeting, we discussed my recent assessment which showed progress in some areas. We discussed my need to reduce multi-tasking and learn better priotitizing skills. Then we discussed their upcoming talk about the connection between exercise, blood flow, and brain health, which really captured my attention, The talk will be posted on their site as a resource in two or three weeks. Great coach! Very encouraging.

The interface with the program is simple and easy to navigate. They unlock a section after you complete each succeeding one, in order. Also, the next module will not be unlocked until the next day. This can be a little frustrating if you're like me and you miss a few days and want to catch up.

I'm guessing there are some psychological reasons for denying that kind of access so people can't game the system.

Here's a screenshot of the site's dashboard.

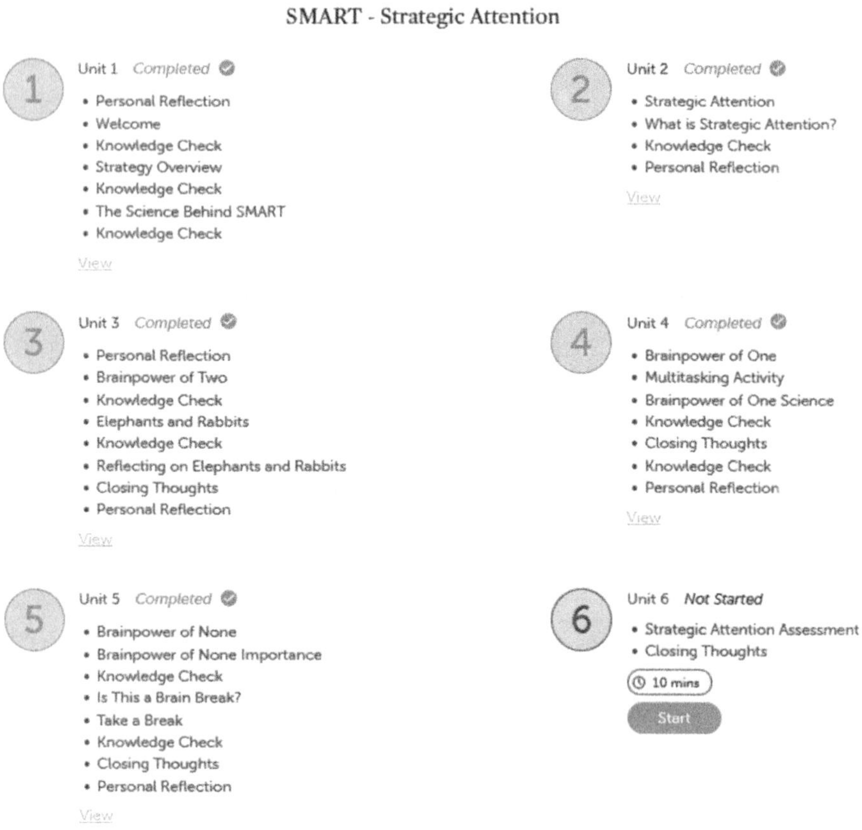

SMART - Strategic Attention

1 Unit 1 *Completed* ✅
- Personal Reflection
- Welcome
- Knowledge Check
- Strategy Overview
- Knowledge Check
- The Science Behind SMART
- Knowledge Check

View

2 Unit 2 *Completed* ✅
- Strategic Attention
- What is Strategic Attention?
- Knowledge Check
- Personal Reflection

View

3 Unit 3 *Completed* ✅
- Personal Reflection
- Brainpower of Two
- Knowledge Check
- Elephants and Rabbits
- Knowledge Check
- Reflecting on Elephants and Rabbits
- Closing Thoughts
- Personal Reflection

View

4 Unit 4 *Completed* ✅
- Brainpower of One
- Multitasking Activity
- Brainpower of One Science
- Knowledge Check
- Closing Thoughts
- Knowledge Check
- Personal Reflection

View

5 Unit 5 *Completed* ✅
- Brainpower of None
- Brainpower of None Importance
- Knowledge Check
- Is This a Brain Break?
- Take a Break
- Knowledge Check
- Closing Thoughts
- Personal Reflection

View

6 Unit 6 *Not Started*
- Strategic Attention Assessment
- Closing Thoughts

🕐 10 mins

Start

In addition to the regular curriculum, you are given opportunities to feed your brain from a selection of written articles and videos as illustrated below.

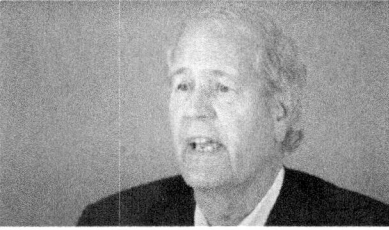

ENGAGED IN LIVING: STORIES OF ALZHEIMER'S

Meaningful Engagement

Who you are doesn't change with a diagnosis of Alzheimer's. Choosing a positive mindset is a step forward. Listen as Craig shares how he holds on to his role within his family and how he's discovered newfound purpose.

Center for BrainHealth

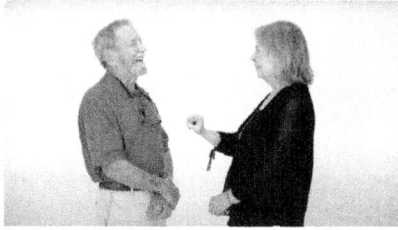

ENGAGED IN LIVING: STORIES OF ALZHEIMER'S

Focusing on Abilities Versus Losses

Education about Alzheimer's is important, but negative ideas can be overwhelming. Don't focus on WHAT IF. Instead, focus on WHAT IS. Come with Bob and Annette as they share how a change in mindset revealed so much to be thankful for.

Center for BrainHealth

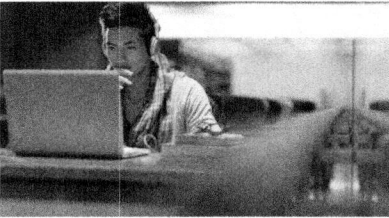

PUBLISHED RESEARCH

Beta and Gamma Binaural Beats Enhance Auditory Sentence Comprehension

Tuesday, February 28, 2023

Growing research suggests binaural beats can enhance brain performance and feelings of well-being, including this study investigating the impact of binaural beat stimulation on complex sentence comprehension and awareness of morpho-syntactic errors.

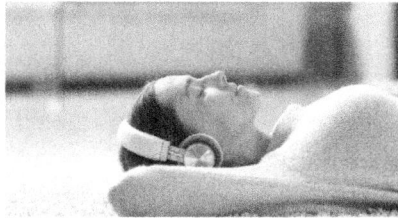

NEWS COVERAGE

Focus on the Arts: This is Your Brain on Music

Friday, February 24, 2023

Why does Vivaldi nourish Bonnie Pitman's brain? The former Dallas Museum of Art director chats with WRR about the impact of music, art and BrainHealth Week to engage "the playful brain, the intellectual brain, the artistic brain."

WRR Classical 101

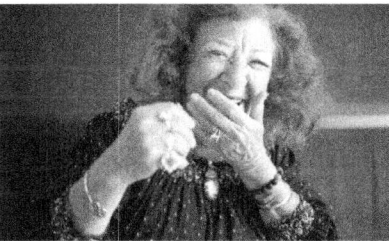

KNOW BRAINERS: BRAIN-HEALTHY TIPS

Laugh to Light up Your Brain

Connecting with a good joke activates the brain's pleasure-and-reward center, elevating endorphins, dopamine and serotonin, a powerful mood-regulating neurotransmitter.

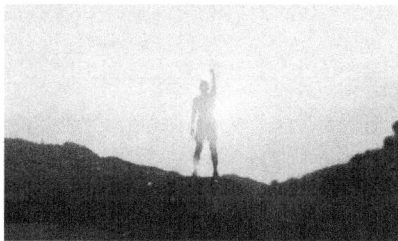

KNOW BRAINERS: BRAIN-HEALTHY TIPS

Make Stress Reduction Your Superpower

Call upon practical, science-driven tools to dial down stress and anxiety. Simple, proven steps can lower stress and strengthen your brain's capacity for reason.

It's impossible to show you the richness of resources available through the BrainHealth Project in this short chapter, but you'll get an idea here

Below is a diagram explaining part of the SMART curriculum. They have put three decades and millions of dollars into this study and it can be an invaluable resource in your journey toward brain health.

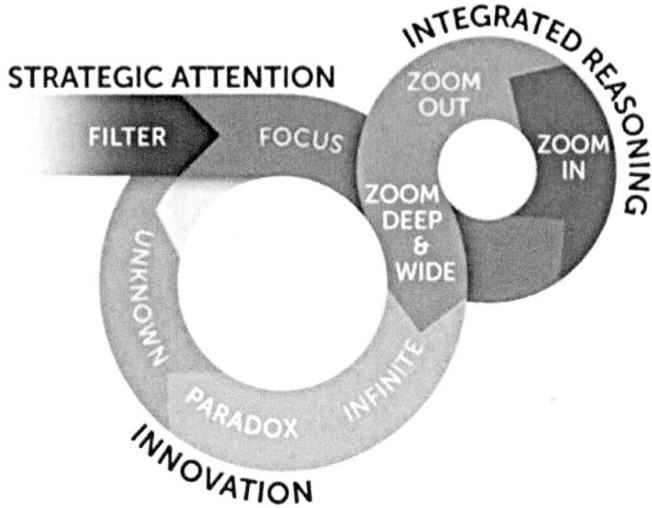

If you're interested, just visit their websites.

The Center for BrainHealth -

https://centerforbrainhealth.org/

The BrainHealth Project -

https://platform.thebrainhealthproject.org/

14

The Diet and Nutrition Wars
Where the food hits the fan!

If you're new to the study of diet and nutrition, you might not be aware of the raging battles between various food tribes: vegan vs meat eaters, Mediterranean vs Paleo, low fat vs low carb, *Calories Don't Count* vs *Oh Yes They Do!** It's an intense battle with wildly conflicting claims and confusing skirmishes over obscure and arcane nutrients. It's hard to determine just what a person should believe or not believe.

Many years ago I read a book titled *Telling Lies for Fun and Profit* by Lawrence Block. That's a clever title for a how-to book on writing fiction professionally. Imagine my surprise when I discovered that a lot of people in the diet and nutrition field are using Block's playbook in the guise of nonfiction, and some of them have an MD or PhD after their name! *Telling Nutrition Lies for Fun and Profit*! This, of course, makes everything even harder to figure out.

What's a person to do? And does it really make any difference, since, as everyone knows —

All Diets Work
and then
All Diets Fail (almost)

Solid figures are hard to come by in the diet and weight loss field, but I asked an AI program about this and they cited a study from UCLA. Traci Mann, PhD, a UCLA associate professor of psychology and the lead author of the study, said, *"We found that the majority of people regained all the weight, plus more."* She went on quantify that for us. "People on diets typically lose 5 to 10 percent of their starting weight in the first six months, however, at least one-third to two-thirds of people on diets regain more weight than they lost within four or five years." Among those who were followed for fewer than two years, 23 percent gained back more weight than they had lost, while of those who were followed for at least two years, 83 percent gained back more weight than they had lost. One study, Mann said, found that five years after the diet, half of the dieters *gained more than 11 pounds over their starting weight.* And the depressing news just keeps on coming.

"Several studies indicate that dieting is actually a consistent predictor of future weight gain," said Janet Tomiyama, a UCLA graduate student and co-author of the study. One study found that both men and women who participated in formal weight-loss programs gained significantly more weight over a two-year period than those who had not participated in a weight-loss program. I think what they're saying is, "If you want to lose weight, don't join a weight loss program." What's a person to do?

And yes, your diet is crucial to your health, so let's look at another study that paints a different picture. A large group of doctors, from some of the top medical schools around the world, studied the dietary habits of people in countries around the world over a period of 27 years and published the results in the Lancet in 2017 as "Health effects of dietary risks in 195 countries, 1990–2017: a systematic analysis for the Global Burden of Disease Study." Behind that exquisitely boring title is some interesting, dare I say even exciting, news — **what we *don't eat* is killing us.**

The first line of the article sets out the basic concept: *"Suboptimal diet* is an important preventable risk factor for non-communicable diseases." In other words, the major causes of death in the world are non-communicable diseases — we don't catch fatal diseases from other people, we give them to ourselves, largely through our suboptimal (poor, deficient, delicious, crappy) diets. They calculated that 11 million people in the studied populations died needlessly between 1990 and 2017 simply from *not eating* certain things.

Before I reveal this miracle manna from Heaven that can extend your life, let me mention that there are four things listed in the study that we eat too much and we will list these separately later. Here are the various types of diets that can extend your life, in order, by number of lives saved:

1. Diets high in whole grains
2. Diets high in fruits
3. Diets high in nuts and seeds
4. Diets high in vegetables
5. Diets high in seafood (omega 3)
6. Diets high in fiber
7. Diets high in polyunsaturated fatty acids
8. Diets high in legumes
9. Diets high in calcium
10. Diets high in milk

Are you surprised at this list? What about the foods we should be eating less, the ones that are shortening our lives?

1. Diets high in salt (sodium – It's really, really bad.)
2. Diets high in sugar-sweetened beverages
3. Diets high in processed red meat
4. Diets high in red meat

I'll have to admit I was a little surprised at the order of items, but not the overall picture they present. Speaking of pictures, here's one you probably saw back in the 70s.

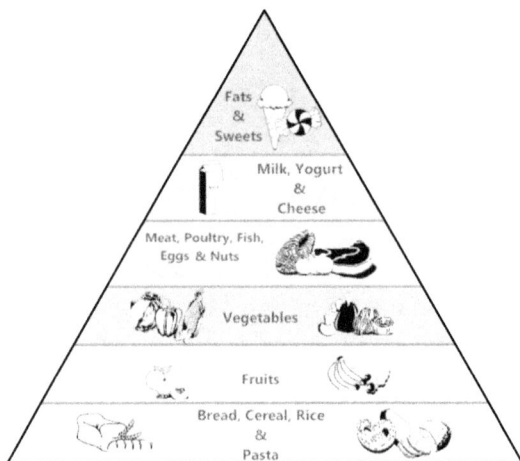

Yes, it's the USDA food pyramid. Some things changed over the years: the breads, cereals and pasta are now all *whole grain*, and the rice is now *brown* rice. Red meat has moved way up and dairy moved up some. About four decades later, the food pyramid morphed into the "Food Plate." Almost all developed countries have something similar. So the takeaway message from the big 27-year, 195 country study is, "Hey, we weren't kidding with the food pyramid thing — follow it or die!"

Before we go any further, I need to disclose some information about me. I am an *omnivore*. I eat all kinds of stuff — the good, the bad, and the deliciously ugly! Is this the best diet? The healthiest? Oh no, far from it. I'm convinced, based upon the best evidence, that a plant-dominant, whole-food diet is unquestionably the best and the healthiest. It's just that I'm a *human*! You know, a flawed, weak, paving-the-road-to-hell-with-good-intentions human. I'll bet you know what I'm talking about. Almost all diets look like this to me:

1. Make a list of all the foods you like.

2. Don't eat 'em.

3. You're welcome!

That's why I keep slipping into the default diet of most people. The apostle Paul described it pretty clearly a couple thousand years ago:

The St. Paul Diet

I do not understand what I eat. For what I want to eat , I do not eat, but what I don't want to eat, I eat. I have the desire to eat what is good, but I cannot carry it out. Now if I eat what I do not want to eat, it is no longer I who does it, but it is the Devil who makes me do it.

Adapted from Romans 7: 15-20 (with apologies to St. Paul, King James, and others).

It's sort of a semi-halfway, backslider's plant-based, sometimes, maybe, diet.

OK, back to the food pyramid/plate. Did you notice that most of the things on the "good for living longer" list are carbohydrates? And the "bad for you" list includes salt, sugar and *red meats*? This is important because there is a current surge of interest in low-carb, high meat and animal fat diets that include the Carnivore Diet, the Keto Diet, the Paleo Diet, the Proper Human Diet, and others.

A diet high in fiber is more important for longevity than a diet low in carbohydrates.
Nir Barzilai, *Age Later*

These diets (often including supplements sold by the same people) are promoted on social media by doctors, some of whom lack credentials. One doctor, who is prominent on YouTube, runs a small-town family medicine practice. He routinely criticizes MD and PhD nutrition science professors and molecular biologists who have published many nutrition focused peer-reviewed, papers in medical journals. This doctor even posted on YouTube, a video of himself at the drive-through window of a McDonald's, ordering "seven quarter-pound hamburger patties stacked up in a container." He then proceeds to pick up a patty with his fingers "like a true carnivore" he says, and eats a chunk of it. A robust display of manliness that comes from eating meat, no doubt. This small town quarter-pound-burger-eating doctor serves as a *nutritional* guru to 3.7 *million followers* on YouTube. Unbelievable! (More transparency: I have eaten chicken-fried bacon. On purpose. That's bacon that has been coated with breading then deep fried. *Mea Culpa!* Yes, *I am* that stupid, but I didn't put it on YouTube as a display of my nutritional smartness.)

There is a glaring problem with all of these low-carb, meat-centric diets — they recommend that you *do not eat* any of the foods listed in the big study as life-extending! They are all *completely* sub-optimal and the star of their diets is red meat, which only appears on the *life-shortening list* in that study.

The Carnivore Diet, yeah, that's the ticket!

In a world obsessed with fad diets and quick fixes, the carnivore diet stands out as a beacon of absurdity. Proponents of this meat-centric regimen tout its supposed benefits, claiming it leads to rapid weight loss and improved health. But scratch beneath the surface, and you'll find a recipe for disaster—a diet devoid of essential nutrients, lacking in fiber, and ultimately detrimental to long-term well-being.

Let's start with the glaring issue: fiber deficiency. The carnivore diet, as the name suggests, revolves around the consumption of animal products exclusively. This means waving goodbye to fruits, vegetables, grains, and all other sources of fiber—the very substance that keeps our digestive system humming along smoothly. Without fiber, our gut microbiota are left starving for sustenance, leading to constipation, bloating, and a host of other gastrointestinal woes. (If you really want to know more about fiber and your gut, read *Fiber Fueled* by Will Bulsiewicz, a board certified gastroenterologist and gut health expert. It contains a lot of information presented in an easy-to-understand manner.)

While proponents of the carnivore diet may argue that humans can thrive on meat alone, the evidence suggests otherwise. Take a look at the "Blue Zones," regions of the world where people live the longest and healthiest lives. Nowhere in these longevity hotspots will you find a population subsisting solely on steak and bacon. Instead, these centenarians attribute their longevity to a plant-rich diet, packed with fiber, phytochemicals, and other essential

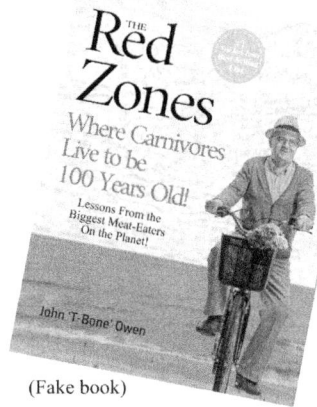

THE Red Zones
Where Carnivores Live to be 100 Years Old!
Lessons From the Biggest Meat-Eaters On the Planet!
John 'T-Bone' Owen

(Fake book)

nutrients. Did you notice that there are no "Red Zones" populated with 100-year-old meat-eaters?

> "Those who ate less meat and more vegetables had less diabetes, less hypertension, less cancer and lower overall mortality."
>
> Nir Barzilai, *Age Later*

Speaking of nutrients, let's talk protein and fiber. While it's true that *very* few Americans are deficient in protein intake, a staggering 97% fall short when it comes to their intake of even the *minimum* recommended amount of fiber. This glaring imbalance speaks volumes about the priorities of our modern diet culture. We're so fixated on protein that we've neglected the humble fiber—the unsung hero of digestive health.

And what about phytochemicals? These potent plant compounds play a crucial role in protecting against chronic diseases, yet they're virtually absent from the carnivore diet. Incidentally, phytochemicals means plant chemicals. Instead, carnivores load up on saturated fats, a dietary choice that's been linked to atherosclerosis, cardiovascular problems and other health issues. It's like trying to build a house with bricks made of butter—sure, it might hold up for a while, but eventually, it's bound to soften and slump.

But perhaps the most insidious aspect of the carnivore diet is its impact on mental health. The gut-brain connection is well-established, with research suggesting that gut health directly influences mood and cognitive function. Books like *The Second Brain* by Michael Gerson or *The Age Proof Brain,* by Marc Milstein provide a Tsunami of information about the *gut-brain connection.* Yet, by depriving their gut of necessary fiber and nutrition, carnivores are unwittingly sabotaging their mental well-being. Maybe that's why they're so quick to embrace such an extreme diet — they're not thinking straight because of their meat-heavy brain fuel?

The circus of diets that parade through our cultural landscape is a veritable smorgasbord of bizarre ideas and conflicting philosophies. From the carnivore diet to the vegan diet, from low-carb to low-fat, it seems there's a diet for every palate and persuasion. Yet, despite their fervent promises of success, the sad truth is that almost all diets ultimately fail to deliver long-term results. Studies have shown that 90% *or more* of diets end in disappointment, with dieters regaining the weight they lost and often packing on even more pounds in the process as described above. And while some proponents claim that calories don't count—that you can eat whatever you want as long as you stick to certain food groups—just take a look at the famously infamous Twinkie Diet.

The Twinkie Diet

The "Twinkie Diet," sometimes called "The Convenience Store Diet," refers to an experiment conducted by Mark Haub, a nutrition professor at Kansas State University, in 2010. Over a 10-week period, Haub primarily consumed processed snack foods like Twinkies, Oreos, and Doritos every three hours instead of regular meals, while also taking a multivitamin and drinking a protein shake daily. He limited his intake to about 1,800 calories a day, which was less than his usual consumption. Surprisingly, Haub lost 27 pounds during this experiment, and his body mass index (BMI) returned to a normal range. Additionally, his "bad" cholesterol (LDL) decreased by 20%, his "good" cholesterol (HDL) increased by 20%, and his triglycerides decreased by 39%. It's important to note the obvious: this diet was *not* nutritionally balanced or sustainable in the long term. Haub simply wanted to demonstrate that calorie counting and creating a calorie deficit are important factors in weight loss, regardless of the nutritional value of the food consumed.

Sure, you might shed a few pounds subsisting on a diet of processed junk food, but the toll it takes on your health and well-being is hardly worth the temporary slim-down.

Similar to the carnivore diet, the currently popular Paleolithic diet, or paleo diet, centers on the idea that eating like our early ancestors ate aligns with our genetics and promotes good health. It's also known as the caveman, Stone Age, or steak and bacon diet. Basically, it calls for eating mostly meats with few vegetables (carbs) and no sugars or processed foods. Unfortunately, highly informed anthropologists and evolutionary biologists say that the basic premise is flawed because paleo man ate whatever they could get their hands on. Everything from roots, fruits and berries to insects, small rodents, and, yes, *wild* animals (not domesticated, and *no* steak or bacon). Also they lived only 25 to 30 years and were small in stature.

Except for a few people with specific disease conditions, low-carb, meat-centric diets are nothing more than a misguided attempt to hack your way to health. By forsaking a balanced diet with fiber, phytochemicals, and other essential vitamins and minerals, carnivores are playing a dangerous game with their well-being. Instead of reaching for another hamburger patty, perhaps it's time to embrace the wisdom of the Blue Zones and prioritize a balanced, plant-rich diet. Maybe they need to grab a bowl of oatmeal with some blueberries and almond milk!

15

The "Miracle Molecule" Nitric Oxide

"Sex at my age is like trying to shoot pool . . .with a rope."

George Burns, *Wisdom of the 90's*

Every old man on Earth understands George's dilemma, and probably a few old women as well. His problem is, from a physiological perspective, a lack of nitric oxide, or NO. As we said back in chapter three, NO is a remarkable molecule.

NO Cardiovascular Effects

Nitric oxide (NO) serves as a critical regulator of vascular tone, primarily through its potent vasodilatory effects, which contribute to the regulation of blood pressure. Endothelial cells release NO in response to various stimuli, including shear stress and neurotransmitters. This NO immediately diffuses into adjacent vascular smooth muscle cells, where it activates guanylate cyclase, leading to the production of cyclic GMP. The subsequent signaling cascade results in relaxation of vascular smooth muscle cells, leading to vasodilation and a decrease in systemic vascular resistance, ultimately contributing to the maintenance of normal blood pressure levels.

Additionally, nitric oxide exhibits potent anti-inflammatory and anti-atherogenic effects within the cardiovascular system. NO plays a crucial role in maintaining endothelial homeostasis by inhibiting the expression of adhesion molecules such as vascular cell adhesion molecule-1 (VCAM-1) and intercellular adhesion molecule-1 (ICAM-1), thereby preventing the adhesion and infiltration of leukocytes into the vessel wall. (The beginnings of inflammation) Furthermore, NO suppresses the production of pro-inflammatory cytokines and chemokines, thereby mitigating endothelial dysfunction and vascular inflammation, key processes in the initiation and progression of atherosclerosis.

Moreover, nitric oxide plays a pivotal role in inhibiting platelet activation and aggregation, thereby preventing thrombus formation and maintaining vascular patency. NO inhibits platelet adhesion to the endothelium and activation by reducing intracellular calcium levels and blocking key platelet activation pathways. Additionally, NO promotes the breakup of platelet aggregates and inhibits the release of pro-clotting factors from activated platelets, ultimately preventing the formation of arterial clots and reducing the risk of cardiovascular events such as heart attacks and stroke.

Nitric oxide's multifaceted effects on the cardiovascular system, including vasodilation and blood pressure regulation, anti-inflammatory and anti-atherogenic actions, and inhibition of platelet aggregation and thrombus formation, underscore the importance of NO in maintaining vascular health and preventing cardiovascular diseases.

NO Neurological and Neuromodulatory Functions

Nitric oxide (NO) serves a critical role in the communication between neurons in the brain, influencing neurotransmission and synaptic plasticity. When neurons communicate, NO acts as a signaling molecule that can affect the release of neurotransmitters, the chemicals responsible for transmitting signals between neurons. Additionally, NO contributes to synaptic plasticity, which refers to the brain's ability to adapt and change over time in response to experiences. Through its involvement in neurotransmission and synaptic plasticity, NO plays a fundamental role in various cognitive functions, including learning and Memory.

Beyond its role in neurotransmission, nitric oxide exhibits neuroprotective properties, suggesting its potential implications for neurodegenerative diseases. Neurodegenerative diseases, such as Alzheimer's and Parkinson's, involve the progressive degeneration of neurons, leading to cognitive decline and motor impairments. Research suggests that NO may help protect neurons from damage caused by oxidative stress, inflammation, and other harmful processes implicated in neurodegenerative conditions. By promoting neuronal survival and resilience, NO holds promise as a target for therapeutic interventions aimed at slowing the progression of neurodegenerative diseases.

Numerous studies have demonstrated that people with higher levels of fitness or physical activity perform better on cognitive tasks, especially executive or memory functions.
Stillman, Erickson, 2018

In addition to its neuroprotective effects, nitric oxide influences the perception and processing of pain in the nervous system. NO participates in the regulation of pain signals, affecting the transmission of pain messages to the brain and the interpretation of those signals. This regulation of pain perception by NO contributes to both acute body pain, which results from tissue damage or injury such as a bruise or cut, and chronic neuropathic pain, which arises from nerve damage or dysfunction. Understanding the role of NO in pain regulation may offer insights into the development of new therapeutic approaches for managing pain.

Nitric oxide plays diverse roles in neurological function, including its involvement in neurotransmission and synaptic plasticity, its neuroprotective effects with potential implications for neurodegenerative diseases, and its regulation of pain perception. These functions highlight the significance of NO in maintaining brain health and the nervous system.

NO Immune System Regulation

Nitric oxide (NO) plays a crucial role in regulating the immune system's response to pathogens and maintaining host defense mechanisms. One of its primary functions is its antimicrobial activity, where NO acts as a potent antimicrobial agent against a wide range of pathogens, including bacteria, viruses, and parasites. By inhibiting the growth and replication of these pathogens, NO helps the body fend off infections and protect against microbial invaders. Additionally, NO enhances the function of immune cells such as macrophages and white blood cells, which are essential components of the body's innate immune response.

In addition to its direct antimicrobial effects, nitric oxide exerts effects on your immune system's response to inflammatory stimulus, helping to regulate the magnitude and duration of immune reactions. NO can dampen excessive inflammation by suppressing the production of inflammatory cytokines and inhibiting the activation of inflammatory signaling pathways. By regulating the immune response, NO can help clear up inflammation and help the restoration of tissue homeostasis following infection or injury. However, the failure of NO-mediated immunity can lead to immune-related disorders characterized by chronic inflammation.

While nitric oxide plays a crucial role in defending against pathogens and regulating immune responses, it doesn't work right, it can contribute to the development of autoimmune diseases and chronic inflammation. In autoimmune diseases, the immune system mistakenly attacks the body's own tissues, leading to tissue damage and inflammation. NO can contribute to autoimmune problems by promoting the activation of some immune cells that can exacerbate tissue inflammation. Furthermore, excessive production of NO in chronic inflammatory conditions can contribute to tissue damage and promote disease progression.

Nitric oxide serves as a key regulator of the immune system, through antimicrobial activity, regulation of inflammatory responses, and influencing the development of autoimmune diseases and chronic inflammation. While NO plays a critical role in defending against pathogens and maintaining immune homeostasis, the *lack* of NO can contribute to immune-related disorders and inflammatory diseases.

NO In Exercise Physiology and Metabolism

Nitric oxide (NO) plays a pivotal role in exercise physiology and metabolism, exerting various effects on skeletal muscle perfusion, glucose uptake, insulin sensitivity, and mitochondrial biogenesis. One of its primary functions is vasodilation, where NO promotes the relaxation of blood vessels, leading to increased blood flow to skeletal muscles during exercise. This enhanced perfusion delivers oxygen and nutrients to active muscle fibers, increasing energy production and waste removal. Additionally, NO-mediated vasodilation helps regulate blood pressure and maintain cardiovascular function during physical activity.

> **"There may be no better way of keeping your arteries clean and flexible than to maximize your own production of nitric oxide."**
> Louis Ignarro, MD, *NO More Heart Disease*

The vasodilatory effect of NO is what causes blood engorge the penis causing an erection. As we said at the beginning of this chapter, the *lack* of NO is what caused George Burns to experience his "rope syndrome."

In addition to its vasodilation effects, nitric oxide plays a crucial role in regulating glucose uptake and insulin sensitivity in skeletal muscle cells. NO promotes the movement of glucose proteins to the cell membrane, helping the uptake of glucose from the bloodstream into muscle cells. This increased glucose uptake enhances energy availability for muscle contraction and glycogen synthesis, supporting exercise performance and recovery. Furthermore, NO enhances insulin sensitivity by promoting cellular signaling pathways that enhance insulin action, contributing to glucose homeostasis and metabolic health.

Nitric oxide also influences mitochondrial biogenesis and energy metabolism in skeletal muscle cells, contributing to the adaptation to exercise training and endurance performance. NO stimulates the production of mitochondria, the cellular organelles responsible for energy production through oxidative processes. This increase in mitochondrial biogenesis enhances the capacity for aerobic metabolism, allowing muscles to sustain prolonged exercise and delay fatigue. Furthermore, NO regulates mitochondrial function by influencing respiratory chain activity and oxidative stress, optimizing energy production and reducing cellular damage during exercise.

Nitric oxide has a broad role in exercise physiology and metabolism: influencing skeletal muscle perfusion, glucose uptake, insulin sensitivity, and mitochondrial biogenesis. By promoting vasodilation, NO also: enhances blood flow to active muscles, supports energy production and nutrient delivery during exercise, boosts glucose metabolism and mitochondrial function.

NO Versus COVID-19

There is a possibility that reduced endothelial NO production could be a common underlying pathology for the progression of COVID-19. An article by Jun Kobayashi, titled "NO In Exercise Physiology and Metabolism," was published in the journal, *Nitric Oxide in 2022*, explaining how studies of SARS-CoV-2 infection show that *NO inhibits the development of COVID-19*, including (1) virus entry into host cells, (2) viral replication, (3) host immune response, and (4) subsequent blood clot complications. It appears that restoring NO in your body may have the potential to be a preventive or early-treatment option for COVID-19.

The study provides an in-depth discussion of NO to prevent SARS-CoV-2 infection, particularly by focusing on lifestyle factors such as [1] nitrate-rich diets, [2] endurance physical exercise *(such as brisk walking)*, and [3] nasal breathing *(especially Bee Breathing)*, which could be easily performed on a daily basis to boost your NO bioavailability

Did you notice that?

This study, published in a peer-reviewed medical journal, written by a doctor/scientist does NOT recommend a shot or pill, or even a supplement, but a course of ***do-it-yourself steps*** to boost your NO!

R Your Prescription:

1. Eat leafy green vegetables

2. Walk 3 miles daily

3. Hum while exhaling when you walk

16

Exercise and the Hallmarks of Aging

As we age, our bodies undergo various changes that contribute to the development of age-related diseases and a decline in overall health. These changes are often characterized by nine* hallmarks of aging, which include:

1. Genomic instability

2. Telomere attrition

3. Epigenetic alterations

4. Loss of proteostasis

5. Deregulated nutrient sensing

6. Mitochondrial dysfunction

7. Cellular senescence

8. Stem cell exhaustion

9. Altered intercellular communication

While these hallmarks may seem daunting, emerging research suggests that regular exercise has the remarkable ability to improve or mitigate many of these age-related processes, thereby promoting healthier aging.

Research has shown that genomic instability, which refers

---

*There are other studies that propose from seven to twelve hallmarks.

to errors in our DNA, can be attenuated by exercise-induced DNA repair mechanisms. Similarly, exercise has been found to counteract telomere shortening of protective caps at the ends of our chromosomes. Exercise has also been linked to epigenetic changes that regulate gene expression.

> Exercise should be seen as a pill, which improves the
> health-related quality of life and functional capabilities
> while mitigating physiological changes
> and comorbidities associated with aging.
> *Rebelo-Marques, et al, 2018*

The breakdown of protein homeostasis (proteostasis) in cells, is another hallmark of aging that can be positively influenced by exercise. Exercise promotes protein turnover, which is when the body breaks down old proteins into their basic parts (amino acids) and then uses those to make new proteins. Any left over parts are discarded helping to maintain cellular function. Additionally, exercise has been found to control nutrient sensing pathways such as insulin signaling, which can help regulate metabolism and prevent metabolic disorders.

Mitochondrial dysfunction, a hallmark characterized by reduced energy production and oxidative stress, can also be mitigated by exercise. Exercise enhances mitochondrial biogenesis and function, leading to improved energy metabolism. Exercise also releases a cascade of powerful antioxidants leading to reduced oxidative damage. Cellular senescence, the end of cellular divisions, can be improved by exercise-induced anti-inflammatory and antioxidant effects, as observed in several studies.

Exercise has also been shown to counteract stem cell exhaustion, a hallmark associated with decreased regenerative capacity and tissue repair. By promoting the creation and activation of stem cells, exercise can help maintain tissue homeostasis and repair. Finally, altered intercellular communication, which contributes to age-related chronic inflammation, can be modified by exercise-induced changes in immune function and signaling pathways.

Gene instability

Gene instability, characterized by DNA damage and mutations, is a fundamental hallmark of aging. However, emerging evidence suggests that regular exercise can lessen this instability by enhancing DNA repair mechanisms. For instance, research has demonstrated that exercise promotes the activation of DNA repair pathways by cutting out damaged or defective parts, thereby reducing the accumulation of DNA injuries. It was found that individuals engaging in endurance exercise exhibited lower levels of DNA damage by oxidation, a common contributor to gene instability in aging cells.

Telomere attrition

A study investigating the impact of exercise on telomere shortening, a key aspect of gene instability, found that people engaging in regular physical activity exhibited slower telomere shortening rates compared to sedentary people. This finding suggests that exercise may counteract telomere erosion, preserving gene stability and potentially delaying cellular senescence. Similarly, there is a positive correlation between exercise frequency and telomerase activity, an enzyme responsible for telomere maintenance, further demonstrating the protective role of exercise against gene instability.

Researchers explored the effects of exercise on DNA methylation patterns, another aspect of gene instability linked to aging. Their findings indicated that regular exercise was associated with favorable changes in DNA methylation profiles, particularly in genes involved in cellular aging processes. By promoting epigenetic stability, exercise may contribute to maintaining gene integrity and reduce the risk of age-related diseases. Collectively, these studies underscore the potential of exercise as a regulator of gene instability, highlighting its multifaceted benefits for healthy aging.

> **DNA methylation** is like a tiny label that tells our cells which parts of our DNA should be turned on or turned off. It's a bit like putting sticky notes in a book to mark important pages. When certain parts of our DNA are methylated, it means they're switched on or off as the body requires. This process is really important because it helps our cells know what they're supposed to do and when. Just like following a recipe — and remember, your DNA is a collection of recipes for proteins — our cells need instructions to work properly, and DNA methylation helps provide those instructions.

Telomere attrition refers to the progressive shortening of telomeres, the protective caps located at the ends of chromosomes, which occurs with each round of cell division. This shortening is a natural consequence of cellular replication and is intricately linked to the aging process. As telomeres become increasingly shorter, cells experience senescence or apoptosis, contributing to tissue aging and eventual organ dysfunction. The relationship between telomere length and aging has garnered significant attention in scientific research, with telomere attrition emerging as a hallmark of biological aging and a marker for age-related diseases.

A growing body of research has explored the impact of exercise on telomere length and telomerase activity. Telomerase is the enzyme responsible for maintaining telomere length.

Several studies have demonstrated a strong association between regular physical activity and longer telomeres, suggesting that exercise may mitigate telomere shrinkage. For instance, a longitudinal study involving people engaged in moderate-to-vigorous physical activity showed a correlation between higher activity levels and reduced telomere shortening over time. Moreover, individuals participating in endurance-based exercises, such as walking, running or cycling, exhibited greater telomere length compared to sedentary counterparts, indicating a potential protective effect of aerobic exercise against telomere attrition.

Exercise appears to influence telomerase activity, with research indicating that physical activity may increase telomerase expression and function. One study observed elevated telomerase levels in peripheral blood cells following acute aerobic exercise, suggesting a transient increase in telomerase activity in response to physical exertion. Additionally, investigations into the effects of chronic exercise training have revealed enhanced telomerase activity in skeletal muscle tissue, implicating exercise as a modulator of telomerase-mediated telomere maintenance mechanisms. These findings underscore the potential role of exercise in preserving telomere integrity and promoting healthy aging trajectories.

Epigenetic alterations

Gene expression patterns can be influenced significantly by epigenetic modifications, including DNA methylation, histone modifications, and changes in chromatin structure. These modifications play a critical role in regulating which genes are turned on or off without altering the underlying DNA sequence.

DNA Methylation: This process involves the addition of a methyl group to the DNA molecule. DNA methylation generally turns off gene expression when it occurs in gene promoter regions. Methylation alters the DNA's accessibility to transcriptional machinery, thereby silencing gene expression. Changes in methylation patterns are associated with various physiological processes and diseases, including cancer and aging.

Histone Acetylation: DNA winds around histones (a group of eight proteins) to form your chromasomes. Histones are little bundles of eight proteins that serve as spools. The main "thread" of the DNA, the double-helix spiral, wraps around these spools looking sort of like pearls on a chain, before being tightly wound into the big X shape which is called a chomosome. A complex process, known as *acetylation*, weakens the connection between histones and DNA. This leads to a more relaxed, looser DNA structure that promotes transcriptional (talking, writing) activities. Histone acetylation is dynamic and reversible, It plays a key role in regulating which genes get turned or turned off in response to environmental signals.

Exercise has has positive benefits for men
and women at every stage of life.

Chromatin Structure: Chromatin is the DNA and histones that make up your chromasome, which exist in several forms: a tightly packed form called heterochromatin, which is an inactive communicator, or a loosely packed form called euchromatin, which is an active communicator. The structure of chromatin is subject to various post-translational modifications. These modifications can influence the binding of regulatory proteins to the DNA, thereby controlling gene expression .

Exercise and Epigenetic Modulation

Exercise is known to modulate these epigenetic processes, contributing to improvements in health and potentially reversing some age-related changes.

DNA Methylation: Regular physical activity has been

shown to lead to changes in DNA methylation patterns. For example, a study demonstrated that exercise can lead to hypomethylation (reduced methylation) of genes involved in energy metabolism and inflammation. These changes can enhance metabolic efficiency and reduce chronic inflammation, which are crucial for maintaining health during aging .

Histone Modifications: Histones are little bundles of eight proteins that serve as spools. The main "thread" of the DNA, the double-helix spiral, wraps around these spools looking sort of like pearls on a chain, before being tightly wound into the big X shape.Exercise influences how tight these histones are wrapped (histone acetylation), leading to a looser, more open structure with increased expression of beneficial genes. For instance, histone acetylation of genes involved in muscle growth and repair can be increased following physical activity. This modification helps in muscle adaptation and recovery, contributing to overall physical fitness and resilience against age-related decline .

Chromatin Remodeling: Physical activity can induce

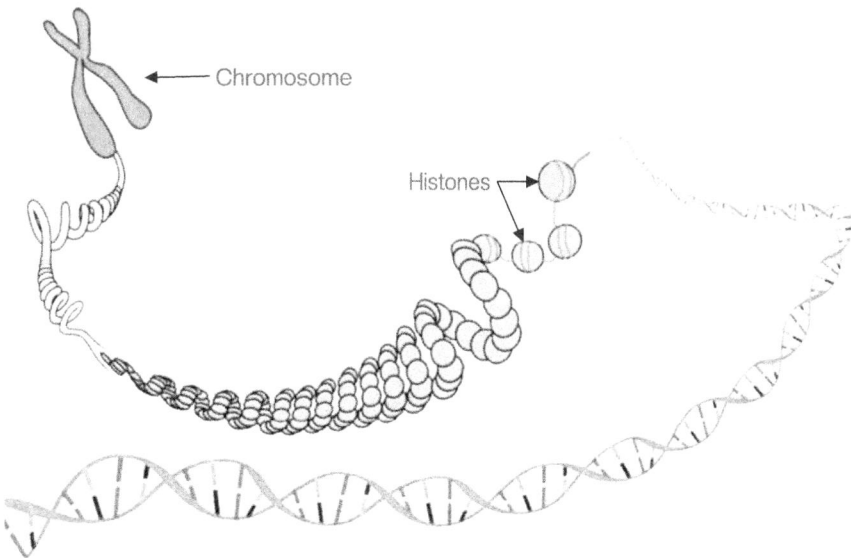

chromatin remodeling, which facilitates the expression of genes important for mitochondrial function, oxidative stress response, and angiogenesis. By promoting the transcription of these genes, exercise helps improve cellular function and adaptability. Such chromatin changes are part of the body's adaptive response to regular physical activity and are beneficial in maintaining cellular health and delaying the onset of age-associated diseases .

In summary, exercise acts as a powerful epigenetic modulator that can positively influence gene expression patterns through changes in DNA methylation, histone acetylation, and chromatin structure. These modifications not only improve overall health but also help mitigate age-related declines, thereby enhancing longevity.

Regular exercise stimulates the machinery in our cells that recycle proteins. This directly targets **impaired proteostasis**, the hallmark of aging characterized by the accumulation of damaged proteins.

Nir Barzilai, *Age Later*

17

Know Your Numbers

*If you don't know where you're going,
when you get there, you're lost.*

Yogi Berra

Goals can be the compass that guide you through any endeavor, providing direction, purpose, and motivation. They are the bridge between your present reality and your desired future, transforming abstract desires into concrete achievements. Goals can serve as a driving force that propels you forward.

The true power of goals, however, lies not in their existence, but in how we use them. Large, overarching goals, while attractive and desirable, can be daunting. This is where your goal-setting becomes crucial. By breaking down your grand visions into smaller, manageable parts with clear, measurable milestones, you create a roadmap to success.

This approach transforms the intimidating into the achievable, the distant into the real. Each small victory becomes a stepping stone, building momentum and confidence as you progress.

As you prepare to "Get fit and live longer," you need to know the specific milestones that will keep you on the path to that ultimate goal. Here are few intermediate markers that will help propel your journey towards your goals while letting you know how you're doing on achieving success.

1. Resting Heart Rate (RHR)

Resting Heart Rate is the number of times your heart beats per minute when you're at complete rest. It's an important indicator of your cardiovascular health and fitness level. A lower RHR generally indicates better cardiovascular fitness and more efficient heart function.

RHR affects physiology by influencing the workload on your heart. A lower RHR means your heart doesn't have to work as hard to pump blood throughout your body, which can lead to improved cardiovascular endurance and potentially a longer lifespan. Studies have shown that a higher RHR is associated with increased risk of cardiovascular disease and all-cause mortality.

To influence your RHR, regular cardiovascular exercise is key. As you become more fit, your heart becomes stronger and more efficient, leading to a lower RHR. Other factors that can help lower RHR include stress reduction techniques like meditation, maintaining a healthy weight, and avoiding tobacco and alcohol.

To measure RHR, simply count your pulse for 60 seconds when you're completely relaxed, preferably in the morning before getting out of bed. Alternatively, many modern fitness trackers and smartwatches can measure RHR automatically. Here's a screenshot of RHR from a FitBit.

2. Body Mass Index (BMI)

Body Mass Index is a simple measure that uses your height and weight to work out if your weight is healthy.

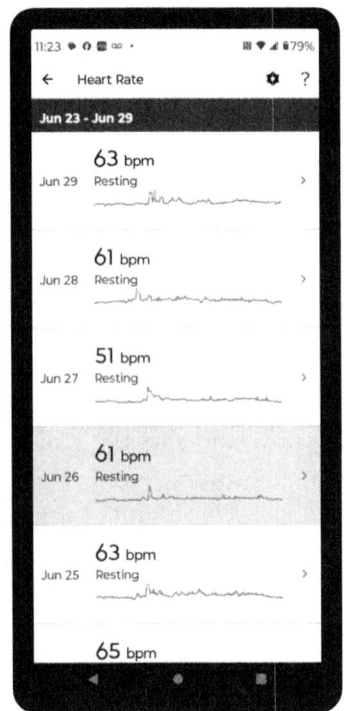

It's an important screening tool used to identify potential weight problems in adults.

BMI affects physiology by providing an indication of body fat content. Higher BMI values are associated with increased risks of various health conditions, including cardiovascular disease, type 2 diabetes, and certain cancers. However, it's important to note that BMI doesn't directly measure body fat and doesn't account for factors like muscle mass, bone density, or overall body composition. To influence your BMI, focus on maintaining a healthy balance between calorie intake and energy expenditure. This typically involves a combination of a balanced diet and regular physical activity. For those looking to lower their BMI, creating a calorie deficit through diet and exercise is key. The formula to calculate BMI is a little complicated. Your body weight divided by your height in inches squared, times a constant of 707. It looks like this:

$$BMI = \frac{180 \ \text{Weight}}{70^2 \ \text{Height Squared}} \quad \frac{180}{4900} = .0367$$

$$.0367 \times \mathbf{707} = \boxed{25.94}$$

This example of a person who weighs 180 pounds and is 70" (5"-10") tall with a BMI of 25.9. A BMI of less that 18.5 is considered thin, from 18,6 to 24.9 is healthy, 25 to 29.9 is overweight, and more than 30 is obese. But, *good news for older people,* those with a BMI of 27 (just a little "fluffy") live longer. A little extra weight can be protective as you age according to Nir Barzilai, director of the aging research programs at Albert Einstein Medical College.

While BMI is a useful tool for population-level health assessments, its relationship with individual longevity is complex. Extremely low and high BMIs are associated with increased mortality risk, while a BMI in the "normal" range (18.5- 25) is generally associated with better health outcomes and longevity.

3. Maximal Oxygen Consumption (VO2 max)

VO2 max, also known as maximal oxygen uptake, is the maximum rate of oxygen consumption measured during incremental exercise. It's considered the gold standard for measuring cardiovascular fitness and aerobic endurance.

VO2 max affects physiology by indicating how efficiently your body can take in, transport, and use oxygen during intense exercise. A higher VO2 max means your body can deliver and use more oxygen, allowing for better endurance and performance in aerobic activities.

To improve your VO2 max, you should engage in regular endurance exercises and, for more fit people, high-intensity interval training (HIIT). Activities like running, cycling, or swimming at varying intensities can help boost your VO2 max over time. Consistency is key, as improvements typically occur over weeks to months of regular training.

Measuring VO2 max typically requires a specialized test in a laboratory setting. The test involves exercising at incrementally higher intensities while wearing a mask that measures oxygen consumption and carbon dioxide production. However, some modern fitness devices provide estimated VO2 max values based on heart rate data and user information.

A higher VO2 max is associated with lower risk of cardiovascular disease and all-cause mortality, potentially contributing to increased longevity. It's an excellent indicator of overall fitness and can be a predictor of health outcomes.

There are many charts about VO2max on the internet. They don't always agree on the numbers. Here's a representative example.

VO$_{2max}$ by Age Group, Performance Level					
Age	Low	Below Average	Above Average	High	Elite
Women					
20-29	<28	28-35	36-40	41-50	≥ 51
30-39	<27	27-33	34-38	39-048	≥ 49
40-49	<26	26-31	32-36	37-46	≥ 47
50-59	<25	25-28	29-35	36-45	≥ 46
60-69	<21	21-24	25-29	30-39	≥ 40
70-79	<18	18-21	22-24	25-35	≥ 36
≥ 80	<15	15-19	20-22	23-29	≥ 30
Men					
18-19	<38	38-45	46-49	50-47	≥ 50
20-29	<36	36-42	43-48	49-55	≥ 56
30-39	<35	35-39	40-45	46-52	≥ 53
40-49	<34	34-38	39-43	44-51	≥ 52
50-59	<29	29-25	36-40	41-49	≥ 50
60-69	<25	25-29	30-35	36-45	≥ 46
70-79	<21	21-24	25-29	30-40	≥ 41
≥ 80	<18	18-22	23-25	26-35	≥ 36

4. Maximum Heart Rate (MHR)

Maximum Heart Rate is the highest number of times your heart can contract in one minute. It's an important metric for designing exercise programs and monitoring exercise intensity. MHR affects physiology by setting the upper limit for cardiovascular exertion. During intense exercise, as you approach your MHR, your heart is working at its maximum capacity to deliver oxygen-rich blood to your muscles. Understanding your MHR helps in designing safe and effective exercise routines.

While you can't significantly change your MHR (it naturally decreases with age), you can use it to guide your exercise intensity. By working out at specific percentages of your MHR, you can target different training zones for various fitness goals.

The most accurate way to determine MHR is through a maximal exercise test conducted by a healthcare professional. However, there are formulas to estimate MHR:

1. The traditional formula: MHR = 220 – your age.
   For a person 65 for example, it's 220-65 = **155**
2. A more recent formula: MHR = 208 - (0.7 × age)
   For a person 65 it's 208-45.5 = **162.5**

These formulas provide estimates and actual MHR can vary significantly between individuals. While MHR itself doesn't directly impact longevity, using it to guide appropriate exercise intensity can contribute to overall cardiovascular health and potentially increased lifespan. Regular exercise at appropriate intensities based on your MHR can improve heart health, reduce the risk of cardiovascular disease, and contribute to better quality of life as you age.

5. Heart Rate Recovery (HRR)

Heart Rate Recovery refers to how quickly your heart rate returns to its resting state after intense exercise. It's an important indicator of cardiovascular health and fitness. HRR reflects the efficiency of your autonomic nervous system, particularly the balance between sympathetic (fight-or-flight) and parasympathetic (rest-and-digest) activity. A faster HRR indicates better cardiovascular fitness and a more efficient autonomic nervous system.

To improve your HRR, focus on regular cardiovascular exercise, particularly high-intensity interval training (HIIT). This type of training challenges your cardiovascular system and can lead to improvements in HRR over time. Additionally, practices that promote relaxation and parasympathetic activation, such as deep breathing exercises or meditation, may also help.

Heart Rate Recovery

Great ....30 or higher
Good 20-29
Average 14-19
Fair 12-13
Poor ....Less than 12

To measure HRR, record your heart rate immediately after intense exercise and again after one minute of rest. The difference between these two numbers is your one-minute HRR. A recovery of 20 beats or more is generally considered good, while less than 12 beats may indicate decreased fitness.

A better HRR is associated with lower risk of cardiovascular disease and all-cause mortality, potentially contributing to increased longevity. It's a valuable metric for tracking improvements in cardiovascular health over time.

6. Waist-to-Hip Ratio (WHR)

Waist-to-Hip Ratio is a measure of body fat distribution, particularly the amount of fat stored around the waist in comparison to the hips. It's an important indicator of health risk, often considered more accurate than BMI for predicting certain health issues.

WHR affects physiology by indicating the distribution of body fat. A higher WHR suggests more abdominal (visceral) fat, which is associated with increased risk of cardiovascular disease, type 2 diabetes, and certain cancers. This is because visceral fat is metabolically active and can influence hormone function and inflammation in the body.

To improve your WHR, focus on overall weight loss through a balanced diet and regular exercise, particularly exercises that target the core. However, it's important to note that spot reduction of fat is not possible, so overall lifestyle changes are necessary.

To calculate WHR, divide your waist circumference by your hip circumference (W/H). For example, if your waist is 3 inches and your hips are 36 inches, your WHR would be 0.83. Generally, a WHR above 0.9 for men or above 0.85 for women indicates increased health risk.

In terms of longevity, a lower WHR (indicating less abdominal fat) is associated with lower risk of premature death and age-related diseases. Maintaining a healthy WHR throughout life can contribute to better health outcomes and potentially increased lifespan.

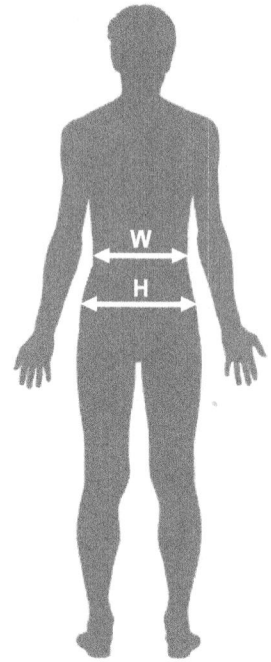

7. Blood Pressure (Systolic/Diastolic)

Blood pressure is the force of blood pushing against the walls of your arteries as your heart pumps blood. It's measured in two numbers: systolic (pressure when the heart beats) and diastolic (pressure when the heart is at rest between beats).

Blood pressure affects nearly every system in the body. Consistently high blood pressure (hypertension) can damage blood vessels, leading to increased risk of heart disease, stroke, kidney problems, and other health issues. On the other hand, very low blood pressure can cause dizziness, fainting, and in severe cases, shock.

To influence your blood pressure, lifestyle modifications are key. These include maintaining a healthy weight, getting regular exercise, especially endurance or aerobic exercise such as walking, jogging, tennis, pickleball and the like. You should also reduce your sodium intake, limit alcohol consumption, manage your stress levels, and you may need medication if prescribed.

Blood pressure is typically measured using a blood pressure device called a sphygmomanometer [really, people, *who comes up with these names?* Some guy named Ralph Sphygmo?], either manually by a healthcare professional or with an automated device you can buy at a drug store.. It's expressed as systolic pressure over diastolic pressure, e.g., 120/80 mmHg. A "normal" blood pressure is usually cited as 130/80, although there is a movement to make it 120/80 or even less.

Whether you are doing it yourself or in your doctors office, you should always: 1) Sit quietly for 5 minutes with your feet flat on the floor. 2) breathe deeply and slowly during this time. 3) Clear your mind of any troubling thoughts. Blood pressure results can vary even over a few minutes. Don't hesitate to ask your doctor/nurse to take it again if you don't like the results. Over the long haul, donating blood regularly can help lower your blood pressure while it offers a much needed resource for people in need of blood transfusions.

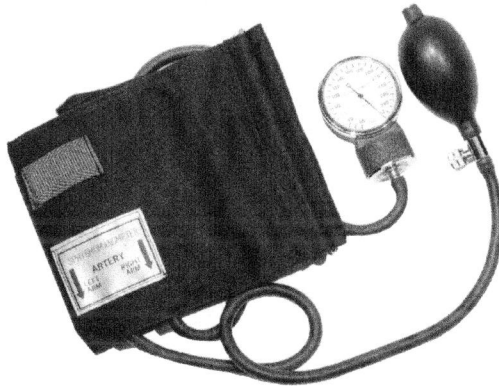

Sphygmomanometer

Maintaining healthy blood pressure is crucial for longevity. Hypertension is a major risk factor for cardiovascular disease, which is a leading cause of death worldwide. In the US, 40% of adults have high blood pressure. For those above 65, a shocking 70% have it. Managing blood pressure effectively can significantly reduce the risk of premature death and disease.

8. C-reactive Protein (CRP)

First, to understand inflammation, we have to understand that inflammation is good. It helps us resolve injuries and protect our bodies from further damage. The problem with inflammation is if injuries and damage do not get resolved, the inflammation turns into *chronic* inflammation. This is bad because high inflammation has been linked to almost all diseases, especially the progressive types such as cancer, diabetes, heart disease, aging, and depression.

C-reactive Protein (CRP) is produced by the liver in response to inflammation in the body. It's an important marker of systemic inflammation and is used to assess risk of cardiovascular disease.

CRP indicates the presence of inflammation, which can be a sign of various health issues including infections, autoimmune disorders, and cardiovascular disease. Chronic low-level inflammation, as indicated by slightly elevated CRP levels, is associated with increased risk of heart disease and potentially other age-related conditions.

To lower CRP levels, you will need to focus on anti-inflammatory lifestyle choices. These include maintaining a healthy weight, regular exercise, following an anti-inflammatory diet rich in whole foods including fruits, vegetables, nuts, and omega-3 fatty acids, while limiting sweets, red meat and processed foods. You should also avoid stress and smoking.

CRP is measured through a blood test ordered by a healthcare provider. There are two types of tests: a regular CRPtest that detects higher levels of the protein, and a high-sensitivity

What do your CRP test results indicate?

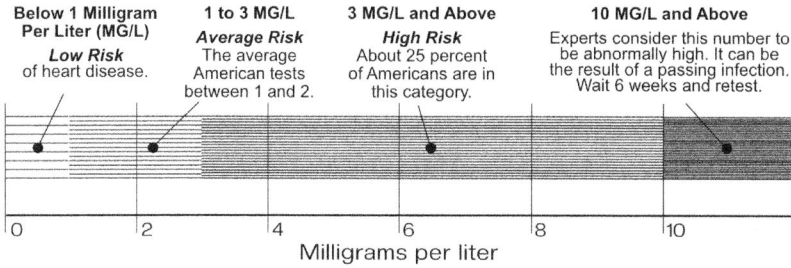

Below 1 Milligram Per Liter (MG/L)	1 to 3 MG/L	3 MG/L and Above	10 MG/L and Above
Low Risk of heart disease.	**Average Risk** The average American tests between 1 and 2.	**High Risk** About 25 percent of Americans are in this category.	Experts consider this number to be abnormally high. It can be the result of a passing infection. Wait 6 weeks and retest.

Milligrams per liter

CRP test (hs-CRP) that can detect lower levels, which is more useful for assessing heart disease risk. A number of places on the internet offer at-home CPR test kits. I'm not sure of their quality, but they may be fine.

In terms of aging and longevity, lower CRP levels are generally associated with better health outcomes and potentially increased lifespan. Chronic inflammation, as indicated by persistently elevated CRP, is thought to contribute to various age-related diseases and accelerated aging.

9. Basal Metabolic Rate (BMR)

Basal Metabolic Rate refers to the number of calories your body burns while at rest to maintain basic life functions. It's a fundamental component of your overall energy expenditure and metabolism.

BMR affects physiology by determining the baseline energy needs of your body. It influences how efficiently your body uses energy from food, which in turn affects weight management, body composition, and overall health. A higher BMR generally means you burn more calories at rest, which can aid in weight management.

To influence your BMR, focus on building and maintaining lean muscle mass through resistance training. Muscle tissue is more metabolically active than fat tissue, so increasing muscle mass can boost BMR. Additionally, staying hydrated, getting adequate sleep, and avoiding extreme calorie restriction (which can lower BMR) are important.

BMR can be estimated using formulas like the Harris-Benedict equation, which takes into account age, gender, height, and weight. For more accurate results, indirect calorimetry tests can be performed in a clinical setting.

While BMR itself doesn't directly impact longevity, maintaining a healthy metabolism through proper nutrition and exercise can contribute to overall health and potentially increased lifespan. A well-functioning metabolism supports healthy weight management and reduces risk factors for various age-related diseases
.

10. Heart Rate Variability (HRV)

Heart Rate Variability is the variation in time between successive heartbeats. It's an important measure of your autonomic nervous system function and overall health.

HRV affects physiology by reflecting the balance between your sympathetic ("fight or flight") and parasympathetic ("rest and digest") nervous systems. Higher HRV generally indicates better cardiovascular fitness, more resilience to stress, and better

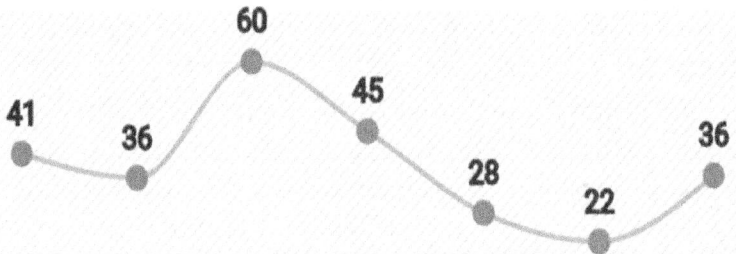

One week HRV as shown on FitBit

overall health. Lower HRV has been associated with increased risk of cardiovascular disease and other health issues.

To improve HRV, focus on stress management techniques such as meditation, deep breathing exercises, and regular physical activity. Adequate sleep, good nutrition, and avoiding excessive alcohol consumption can also positively influence HRV. HRV can be measured using specialized heart rate monitors or some advanced smartwatches and fitness trackers. These devices typically measure HRV over a period of time, often during sleep,

Heart rate variability

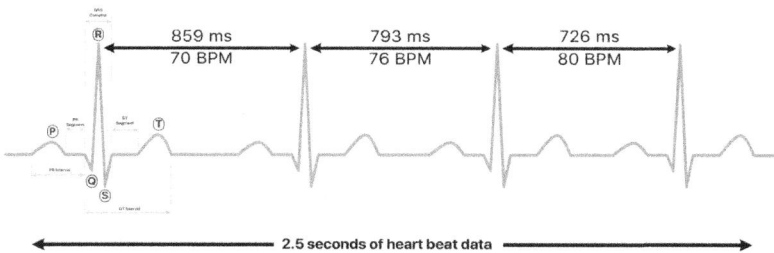

| 859 ms | 793 ms | 726 ms |
| 70 BPM | 76 BPM | 80 BPM |

2.5 seconds of heart beat data

to provide an overall picture of autonomic nervous system function. See FitBit screenshot, on previous page.

In terms of aging and longevity, higher HRV is associated with better health outcomes and potentially increased lifespan. It's considered a marker of biological age and overall health resilience.

11. Blood Glucose Levels (BGL)

Blood Glucose Levels refer to the amount of glucose (sugar) present in your blood. It's a crucial measure for diagnosing and managing diabetes, but it's also important for overall health.

BGL affects physiology by influencing energy availability for cells throughout the body. Consistently high blood glucose levels can damage blood vessels and nerves, leading to various health complications including cardiovascular disease, kidney problems, and neuropathy.

To influence BGL, focus on a balanced diet low in refined carbohydrates and sugars, regular physical activity, and maintaining a healthy weight. For individuals with diabetes, medication may also be necessary to manage blood glucose levels effectively.

BGL can be measured through various methods:

1. Fasting Blood Glucose Test: Measures glucose after an 8-hour fast

2. Random Blood Glucose Test: Measures glucose at any time of day

3. Oral Glucose Tolerance Test: Measures glucose before and 2 hours after drinking a glucose solution

4. Glycated Hemoglobin (HbA1c) Test: Provides an average of blood glucose levels over the past 3 months

Maintaining healthy blood glucose levels is crucial for longevity. Chronically elevated blood glucose, as seen in diabetes, is associated with accelerated aging and increased risk of age-related diseases. Effective blood glucose management can significantly improve health outcomes and potentially increase lifespan.

12. Oxygen Saturation (SpO2)

Oxygen Saturation refers to the percentage of oxygen-saturated hemoglobin relative to total hemoglobin in the blood. It's a crucial measure of how efficiently your body is supplying oxygen to your tissues.

SpO2 affects physiology by indicating how well oxygen is being delivered to your body's cells. Low oxygen saturation can lead to hypoxia, where tissues don't receive enough oxygen, potentially causing organ damage. While you can't directly influence your SpO2 levels, maintaining good overall health can

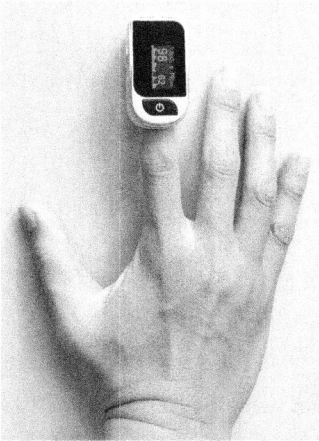

help ensure optimal oxygen saturation. This includes regular exercise to improve lung function, avoiding smoking, and managing any underlying respiratory or cardiovascular conditions.

SpO2 is typically measured using a pulse oximeter, a non-invasive device that clips onto a finger or earlobe. Normal SpO2 levels are generally considered to be between 95-100%.

In terms of aging and longevity, consistently low SpO2 levels can contribute to various health issues and potentially shorten lifespan. Maintaining good oxygen saturation, particularly in older age or with chronic conditions, is important for overall health and longevity.

13. Glycated Hemoglobin (HbA1c)

Glycated Hemoglobin, commonly known as HbA1c, is a form of hemoglobin that is chemically linked to sugar. It provides an average measure of blood glucose levels over the past 3 months. *Glycated* means it has sugar stuck to it. Hemoglobin is the molecule in your red blood cells that sugar sticks to. Since your red blood cells live around 100 days, this sugar will be in your blood for that long. If you are sugar-free for 100 days, your HbA1c should be low, low, low.

HbA1c reflects long-term blood glucose control. Higher levels indicate consistently elevated blood glucose, which can lead to damage of blood vessels and nerves over time. This damage increases the risk of complications such as cardiovascular disease, kidney disease, and neuropathy.

HbA1c (%)	What it means
4.5 - 6.4	Excellent
6.5 - 7.0	Good
7.1 - 8.0	Fair
>80	Poor

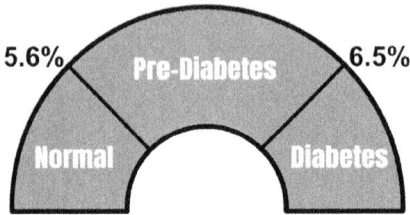

5.6% Pre-Diabetes 6.5%

Normal Diabetes

To influence HbA1c levels, focus on maintaining stable blood glucose levels through a balanced diet, regular physical activity, and weight management. For individuals with diabetes, medication may also be necessary to keep HbA1c within target ranges.

HbA1c is measured through a blood test, usually ordered by a healthcare provider. The result is given as a percentage, with a normal range for non-diabetics typically considered below 5.7%. In terms of aging and longevity, lower HbA1c levels (within the normal range) are associated with better health outcomes and potentially increased lifespan. Effective long-term glucose control, as reflected by HbA1c, can significantly reduce the risk of diabetes-related complications and improve overall health.

There are at-home HbA1c tests available at many drug stores and online. They are moderately priced and reported to be pretty accurate.

14. Total Cholesterol (TC)

Total Cholesterol is the overall amount of cholesterol in your blood, including both "good" (HDL) and "bad" (LDL) cholesterol. It's an important measure of cardiovascular health.

TC affects physiology primarily through its role in atherosclerosis, the buildup of plaque in artery walls (see illustration below, Coronary Artery Disease). While cholesterol is necessary for various bodily functions, excessive levels, particularly of LDL cholesterol, can contribute to cardiovascular disease.

To influence TC levels, focus on a heart-healthy diet low in saturated fats (red meats) and trans fats, engage in regular physical activity, maintain a healthy weight, and avoid smoking. In some cases, medication may be prescribed to help manage cholesterol levels.

Normal Artery   Narrowing of Artery

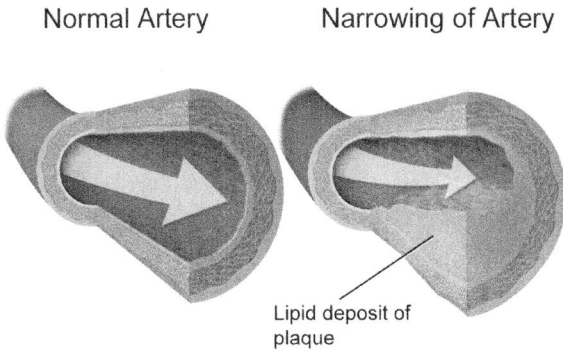

Lipid deposit of plaque

Coronary Artery Disease

TC is measured through a blood test, typically as part of a lipid panel. It's expressed in milligrams per deciliter (mg/dL) or millimoles per liter (mmol/L).

Maintaining healthy cholesterol levels is crucial for longevity. High TC, particularly high LDL cholesterol, is a major risk factor for cardiovascular disease, which significantly impacts lifespan. Managing cholesterol effectively can reduce the risk of heart disease and potentially increase longevity.

15. Low Density Lipoprotein (LDL)

Low Density Lipoprotein, often referred to as "bad" cholesterol, is a type of lipoprotein that carries cholesterol throughout your body. High levels of LDL cholesterol are associated with increased risk of cardiovascular disease.

LDL affects physiology by potentially contributing to the formation of plaque in artery walls (atherosclerosis). This can lead to narrowed or blocked arteries, increasing the risk of heart attack and stroke.

To lower LDL levels, focus on a diet low in saturated and trans fats, high in fiber, and rich in omega-3 fatty acids. Regular physical activity, maintaining a healthy weight, and avoiding smoking are also important. In some cases, medication (like statins) may be prescribed to help lower LDL levels. LDL cholesterol is measured as part of a lipid panel blood test. It's typically expressed in mg/dL or mmol/L.

In terms of aging and longevity, lower LDL levels (within healthy ranges) are associated with reduced risk of cardiovascular disease and potentially increased lifespan. Managing LDL cholesterol effectively is a key strategy for promoting heart health and overall longevity.

16. High Density Lipoprotein (HDL)

High Density Lipoprotein, often called "good" cholesterol, is a type of lipoprotein that helps remove other forms of cholesterol from your bloodstream. Recent research has revealed that *some* HDL proteins are *not* good, but actually contribute to disease states. In studies, an increase in HDL did not affect mortality.

HDL is still good in overall health. It affects physiology by helping to transport excess cholesterol from the body's tissues to the liver for disposal. Higher levels of HDL are generally associated with better cardiovascular health, as it helps protect against the buildup of plaque in the arteries.

To increase HDL levels, engage in regular physical activity, maintain a healthy weight, avoid smoking, and consume a diet based on whole foods and rich in healthy fats (like those found in olive oil, nuts, and fatty fish). .

HDL cholesterol is measured as part of a lipid panel blood test, typically expressed in mg/dL or mmol/L. Higher levels are generally considered beneficial.

In the context of aging and longevity, higher HDL levels (within healthy ranges) are associated with better cardiovascular health and potentially increased lifespan. Maintaining healthy HDL levels, along with managing other lipid parameters, is an important strategy for promoting overall health and longevity.

Why Me, Lord?

What have I ever done to deserve even one of the pleasures I've known?

Kris Kristofferson

I sometimes feel like Kris when I consider the current state of my health and what a miserable job I did of caring for it when I was younger. I ate the Standard American Diet, and I ate a *lot* of it. Plus, I didn't work out very much since I was always *too busy* or *too tired* or something. Maybe you know what that feels like.

But now, you're wondering if you've waited too long to start taking care of your health. The short answer is no. The long answer is noooooo.

In this chapter I'm going to show you my numbers: blood pressure, resting heart rate, VO2max and more. For an old, dad-bodied ordinary man, I have some *extraordinary* numbers, thanks to the amazing ability of the human body to repair itself if you will simply give it a little well-focused attention.

Blood pressure

I'll admit that I'm not very good at taking my own blood pressure. I can take it three times in a row and get three different readings using a battery-operated, wrist-mounted device. It cost around 60 dollars, maybe I should have opted for a more expensive unit. I don't know. At my doctor's office I will sometimes object to the reading. They will retake the test and it will generally be better the second time.

The blood pressure I'm showing here is from my local blood bank when I went in to donate blood. They're always busy and I have plenty of time to sit still, breathe deeply and think calm thoughts — all of which can lower your blood pressure. At any rate my blood pressure at that time was **116 over 69**. Contrast that with what my blood pressure is *supposed* to be.

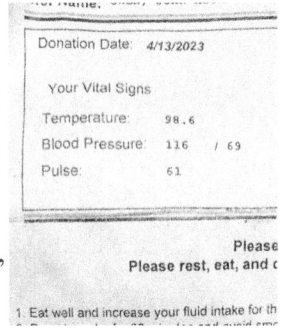

Donation Date: 4/13/2023

Your Vital Signs

Temperature: 98.6
Blood Pressure: 116 / 69
Pulse: 61

Please
Please rest, eat, and c

1. Eat well and increase your fluid intake for th

BLOOD PRESSURE CHART BY AGE

Age	Min	Normal	Max
1 to 12 months	75/50	90/60	110/75
1 to 5 years	80/55	95/65	110/79
6 to 13 years	90/60	105/70	115/80
14 to 19 years	105/73	117/77	120/81
20 to 24 years	108/75	120/79	132/83
25 to 29 years	109/76	121/80	133/84
30 to 34 years	110/77	122/81	134/85
35 to 39 years	111/78	123/82	135/86
40 to 44 years	112/79	125/83	137/87
45 to 49 years	115/80	127/84	139/88
50 to 54 years	116/81	129/85	142/89
55 to 59 years	118/82	131/86	144/90
60 to 64 years	121/83	134/87	147/91
70 TO 79			
80 TO 89		138/90 ?	

Holy cow! I have the blood pressure of a normal teenager—and that's just the beginning. Let's take a look at VO2max which experts in the fitness business generally consider to be the best indicator of cardiovascular fitness and aerobic endurance.

VO2max

We will use the generic figures in the formula for figuring VO2max, then we'll use the actual numbers from my Fitbit.

Calculate VO2max:

Using Formula with Generic Numbers
Max Heart Rate: Constant ÷ Age
220 - 82 = 138

Divided by resting heart rate
138 ÷ 51 = 2.7

2.7 times constant
2.7 x 15.3 = **41**

*Using **Fitbit** Numbers*
Max Heart Rate:
Fitbit=158

158 ÷ by resting heart rate
158 ÷ 51 = 3.09

3.09 x constant
3.09 x 15.3 = **47**

Age	Low	Below Average	Above Average	High	Elite
VO$_{2max}$ by Age Group, Performance Level					
Women					
20-29	<28	28-35	36-40	41-50	≥ 51
30-39	<27	27-33	34-38	39-048	≥ 49
40-49	<26	26-31	32-36	37-46	≥ 47
50-59	<25	25-28	29-35	36-45	≥ 46
60-69	<21	21-24	25-29	30-39	≥ 40
70-79	<18	18-21	22-24	25-35	≥ 36
≥ 80	<15	15-19	20-22	23-29	≥ 30
Men					
18-19	<38	38-45	46-49	50-47	≥ 50
20-29	<36	36-42	43-48	49-55	≥ 56
30-39	<35	35-39	40-45	46-52	≥ 53
40-49	<34	34-38	39-43	44-51	≥ 52
50-59	<29	29-25	36-40	41-49	≥ 50
60-69	<25	25-29	30-35	36-45	≥ 46
70-79	<21	21-24	25-29	30-40	≥ 41
≥ 80	<18	18-22	23-25	26-35	≥ 36

Okay, so I didn't equal a teenager this time, but my numbers are on par with *Elite* athletes 10 to 22 years younger than me, or *Above Average* men 50 years younger!

Resting Heart Rate

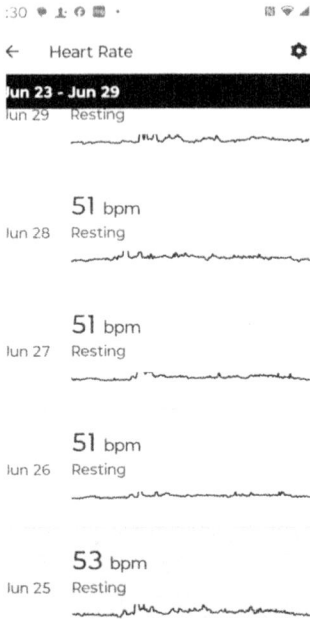

:30 ♥ ⚲ ⊘ ▣ ·   ▨ ⬞ ◢

←   Heart Rate   ✿

Jun 23 - Jun 29
Jun 29   Resting

~~~~~~ᴶᵂᴸᴬ~ᴬ~~~~~~

51 bpm
Jun 28   Resting

~~~~ᴸᴬ~ᴬ~~~~~~~~~

51 bpm
Jun 27   Resting

~~~~~ᵎ ¯~~~~~~~~~~

51 bpm
Jun 26   Resting

~~~~~ᴬ~~~~~~~~~~

53 bpm
Jun 25   Resting

~~~ᴶᴸᴬᴬ~ᴬ~~~~~~~

The Mayo clinic says, "A normal resting heart rate for adults ranges from 60 to 100 beats per minute. Generally, a lower heart rate at rest implies more efficient heart function and better cardiovascular fitness. For example, a well-trained athlete might have a normal resting heart rate closer to 40 beats per minute."

How about that, sports fans? The Mayo Clinic thinks I'm equal to an athlete at any age. What's really funny is that I was *never* equal to an athlete when I was younger!

Several times I have looked at my Fitbit and saw a screen that said my heart rate was 46 at the same time it told me my resting heart rate was 52. Excuse me? To make matters even more confusing, my Fitbit has a screen showing my minimum and maximum heart rate for the day. As you can see from these screenshots, below, taken over several months, the numbers are pretty amazing for a person of any age.

Men: Resting Heart Rate

AGE	18-25	26-35	36-45	46-55	56-65	65+
Athlete	49-55	49-55	50-56	50-57	51-56	50-55
Excellent	56-61	56-61	57-62	58-63	57-61	56-61
Good	62-65	62-65	63-66	64-67	62-67	62-65
Above Average	66-69	66-70	67-70	68-71	68-71	66-69
Average	70-73	71-74	71-75	72-76	72-75	70-73
Below Average	74-81	75-81	76-82	77-83	76-81	74-79
Poor	82+	82+	83+	84+	82+	80+

Heart Rate Variability

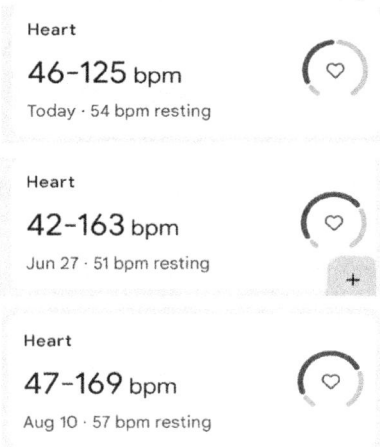

Heart

46-125 bpm

Today · 54 bpm resting

Heart

42-163 bpm

Jun 27 · 51 bpm resting

Heart

47-169 bpm

Aug 10 · 57 bpm resting

I had a hard time finding anything on heart rate variability for a person my age. Actually, you'll notice that most charts exclude data on people above age 65, I finally posed the question to an AI assistant., and here's what it said: "Heart rate variability (HRV) can vary significantly between individuals and is influenced by many factors, including age. HRV typically decreases with age, so what's considered "good" for an 80-year-old man would be different from what's good for a younger adult. For an 80-year-old man, a "good" HRV score would generally be lower than that of a younger adult. One common metric is RMSSD (Root Mean Square of Successive Differences). Based on some studies, for men in their 70s and 80s, an RMSSD value in the range of 15-25 ms might be considered good". I'm not sure how accurate Fitbit is, but several online "experts" think it's pretty accurate. So, if "15 to 25 might be considered good" then what is my 24-to-81 range in one week considered? Remember, with Heart Rate Variablity, *higher is better.*

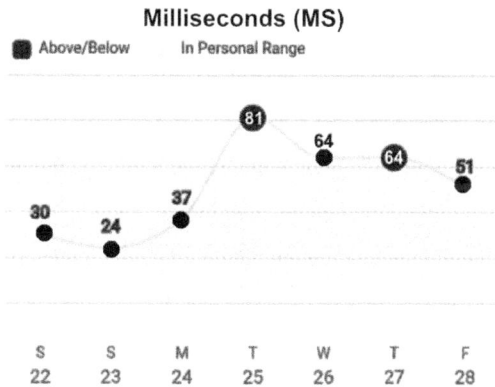

Milliseconds (MS)

■ Above/Below   In Personal Range

81

64

64

51

30

24

37

S   S   M   T   W   T   F
22   23   24   25   26   27   28

Cholesterol A1c

When I enrolled in a Medicare Advantage plan, my new doctor doctor asked if anyone had ever told me that I was pre-diabetic. When I answered no, he said "Well, you are."

The A1c Spectrum

Normal	Pre-Diabetic	Diabetic
5.6 and below	5.7 to 6.4	6.5 and higher

I entered the system at 5.9. When he offered a drug to address the problem, I declined. He said we'd just, "keep an eye on it," and advised that I lose weight, limit sugar consumption and get more exercise.

That's when I began walking — two or three times most weeks, a mile or two each time. I lost two or three pounds. Over the next 15 years my A1c gradually climbed. I walked a little more, cut my daily donuts down to one or two a week. "Maybe it's heredity," he said. Then, 15 years later, I got the dreaded message: I was diabetic. I had breached the 6.5 A1c limit.

This was *not* good news. I was 81, overweight and in moderately dilapidated shape despite visiting the gym semi-occasionally.

This got my attention. Diabetes is serious business and it runs in my family. That's when I decided to see if I could improve my condition. I started walking *every day* aiming for 3.5 miles at 100 paces a minute. Not all at once, but in several shorter walks throughout the day.

My body's first response was to get plantar fasciitis! I visited a Chinese foot massage parlor which was more therapeutic than I could have imagined, then I resumed walking. Gradually, it became easier and bouts of faciitis became less frequent.

I also got a little more serious about my diet. Zero donuts!

Six months later when I had my next exam, the doctor was surprised. I had lost 15 pounds and my A1c had gone from 6.5 to

5.6. I was *not* diabetic, *not* pre-diabetic, but a *normal*, non-diabetic! Was my "genetic problem" a rationalization for my half-hearted attempts to get healthier? Ummm, very likely!

My plan now is to stay healthy by walking, exercising and eating healthier food. Our bodies are remarkably capable of self-repair and maintenance if we will only pay attention to what it truly needs: proper nutrition, physical activity, and social interaction with your fellow humans.

***

As I have said before, I don't come from an exceptional gene pool — just the opposite, in fact. My reason for including these numbers in the book is not to toot my own horn, it's to make the point that even an ordinary old man from a mediocre gene pool who did a poor job of living a healthy life can wind up with good numbers. Meaning that *maybe you can too*!

I genuinely believe that the amazingly powerful things in this book about blood flow, walking, shear stress, mechano-transduction, myokines, a whole food plant-based diet, Klotho, and all the rest hold the keys to improving your numbers. Your improved numbers, of course, are the keys to having a longer, healthier, more vibrant and enjoyable life. That's not a bad tradeoff, and it just might work for you, too. I hope so.

Remember these three things:

1. Exercise *walking, dancing, pickleball, whatever*

2. Eat right *not too much, mostly plants*

3. Socialize *every chance you get*

REFERENCES

Author's note: I suffered a computer disaster while quite far along in this project and lost a great deal of data including many references and my master reference list. Deeply depressed, I went to an AI program, Claude,ai, loaded a chapter into it asking it to come up with references. It did an outstanding job, so I put the rest of the book in. This is the list provided. While not the source material from which I wrote, it is a good resource for those seeking further information on the subject.

Chapter 2

For basic cardiovascular physiology and blood flow:

Hall, J. E., & Hall, M. E. (2020). Guyton and Hall Textbook of Medical Physiology (14th ed.). Elsevier.

For information on mechanotransduction and shear stress:

Davies, P. F. (2009). Hemodynamic shear stress and the endothelium in cardiovascular pathophysiology. Nature Reviews Cardiology, 6(1), 16-26.

For the discovery of nitric oxide and its role in cardiovascular health:

Ignarro, L. J. (2002). Nitric oxide as a unique signaling molecule in the vascular system: a historical overview. Journal of Physiology and Pharmacology, 53(4), 503-514.

For the effects of exercise on nitric oxide production:

Green, D. J., Maiorana, A., O'Driscoll, G., & Taylor, R. (2004). Effect of exercise training on endothelium-derived nitric oxide function in humans. The Journal of Physiology, 561(1), 1-25.

For arteriogenesis and angiogenesis in response to exercise:

Prior, B. M., Yang, H. T., & Terjung, R. L. (2004). What makes vessels grow with exercise training? Journal of Applied Physiology, 97(3), 1119-1128.

For the effects of walking on brain health and hippocampus size:

Erickson, K. I., Voss, M. W., Prakash, R. S., Basak, C., Szabo, A., Chaddock, L., ... & Kramer, A. F. (2011). Exercise training increases size of hippocampus and improves memory. Proceedings of the National Academy of Sciences, 108(7), 3017-3022.

For the role of BDNF in exercise-induced brain plasGcity:

Cotman, C. W., & Berchtold, N. C. (2002). Exercise: a behavioral intervenGon to enhance brain health and plasGcity. Trends in Neurosciences, 25(6),

295-301.

For the concept of "use it or lose it" in brain health:

Höṇ ng, K., & Röder, B. (2013). Beneficial effects of physical exercise on neuroplasticity and cogniҀon. Neuroscience & Biobehavioral Reviews, 37(9), 2243-2257.

For information on myokines and their role in exercise benefits:

Pedersen, B. K., & Febbraio, M. A. (2012). Muscles, exercise and obesity: skeletal muscle as a secretory organ. Nature Reviews Endocrinology, 8(8), 457-465.

For the effects of exercise on Irisin and Klotho:

Severinsen, M. C. K., & Pedersen, B. K. (2020). Muscle—Organ Crosstalk: The Emerging Roles of Myokines. Endocrine Reviews, 41(4), 594-609.

Chapter 3

For the general benefits of walking:

Murphy, M. H., Nevill, A. M., Murtagh, E. M., & Holder, R. L. (2007). The effect of walking on fitness, fatness and resting blood pressure: a meta-analysis of randomised, controlled trials. Preventive Medicine, 44(5), 377-385.

For the study on brief bursts of physical acҀvity:

Stamatakis, E., Huang, B. H., Maher, C., Thogersen-Ntoumani, C., Stathi, A., Dempsey, P. C., ... Hamer, M. (2021). Untapping the health enhancing potential of vigorous intermittent lifestyle physical activity (VILPA): rationale, scoping review, and a 4-pillar research framework. Sports Medicine, 51(1), 1-10.

For the Theory of Effort MinimizaҀon in Physical AcҀvity (TEMPA):

Cheval, B., Radel, R., Neva, J. L., Boyd, L. A., Swinnen, S. P., Sander, D., & BoisgonҀer, M. P. (2018). Behavioral and neural evidence of the rewarding value of exercise behaviors: a systematic review. Sports Medicine, 48(6), 1389-1404.

For the "silly walking" study:

Faulkner, S. H., Rocha, N. R., & Brooker, G. A. (2022). Quantifying the energy expenditure of "inefficient walking": A comparative analysis of 'The Ministry of Silly Walks'. BMJ Open Sport & Exercise Medicine, 8(4), e001479.

For Nordic walking benefits:

Tschentscher, M., Niederseer, D., & Niebauer, J. (2013). Health benefits of Nordic walking: a systematic review. American Journal of Preventive Medicine, 44(1), 76-84.

For walking and cardiovascular health:

Murtagh, E. M., Murphy, M. H., & Boone-Heinonen, J. (2010). Walking: the first steps in cardiovascular disease prevention. Current Opinion in Cardiology, 25(5), 490-496.

For walking and metabolic health:

Hamasaki, H. (2016). Daily physical activity and type 2 diabetes: A review. World Journal of Diabetes, 7(12), 243-251.

For walking and mental health:

Robertson, R., Robertson, A., Jepson, R., & Maxwell, M. (2012). Walking for depression or depressive symptoms: a systematic review and meta-analysis. Mental Health and Physical Activity, 5(1), 66-75.

For walking and joint health:

White, D. K., Tudor-Locke, C., Felson, D. T., Gross, K. D., Niu, J., Nevitt, M., ... & Neogi, T. (2013). Walking to meet physical activity guidelines in knee osteoarthritis: is 10,000 steps enough? Archives of Physical Medicine and Rehabilitation, 94(4), 711-717.

For walking and cognitive function:

Kramer, A. F., Erickson, K. I., & Colcombe, S. J. (2006). Exercise, cognition, and the aging brain. Journal of Applied Physiology, 101(4), 1237-1242.

Chapter 4

For Nrf2 and KLF2 roles in oxidative stress:

Ma, Q. (2013). Role of nrf2 in oxidative stress and toxicity. Annual Review of Pharmacology and Toxicology, 53, 401-426.

SenBanerjee, S., Lin, Z., Atkins, G. B., Greif, D. M., Rao, R. M., Kumar, A., ... & Jain, M. K. (2004). KLF2 Is a novel transcriptional regulator of endothelial proinflammatory activation. The Journal of Experimental Medicine, 199(10), 1305-1315.

For oxidative stress and its effects on the body:

Pizzino, G., Irrera, N., Cucinotta, M., Pallio, G., Mannino, F., Arcoraci, V., ... & Bitto, A. (2017). Oxidative stress: harms and benefits for human health. Oxidative Medicine and Cellular Longevity, 2017.

Sies, H., Berndt, C., & Jones, D. P. (2017). Oxidative stress. Annual Review of Biochemistry, 86, 715-748.

For antioxidants (SOD, GPx, CAT) and their roles:

Ighodaro, O. M., & Akinloye, O. A. (2018). First line defence antioxidants-superoxide dismutase (SOD), catalase (CAT) and glutathione peroxidase (GPX): Their fundamental role in the entire antioxidant defence grid. Alexandria

Journal of Medicine, 54(4), 287-293.

Fukai, T., & Ushio-Fukai, M. (2011). Superoxide dismutases: role in redox signaling, vascular function, and diseases. Antioxidants & Redox Signaling, 15(6), 1583-1606.

For shear stress and KLF2 activation:

Dekker, R. J., van Soest, S., Fontijn, R. D., Salamanca, S., de Groot, P. G., VanBavel, E., ... & Horrevoets, A. J. (2002). Prolonged fluid shear stress induces a distinct set of endothelial cell genes, most specifically lung Krüppel-like factor (KLF2). Blood, 100(5), 1689-1698.

Parmar, K. M., Larman, H. B., Dai, G., Zhang, Y., Wang, E. T., Moorthy, S. N., ... & García-Cardeña, G. (2006). Integration of flow-dependent endothelial phenotypes by Kruppel-like factor 2. The Journal of Clinical Investigation, 116(1), 49-58.

For Nrf2-Keap1 interaction and antioxidant response:

Suzuki, T., & Yamamoto, M. (2015). Molecular basis of the Keap1–Nrf2 system. Free Radical Biology and Medicine, 88, 93-100.

Tonelli, C., Chio, I. I. C., & Tuveson, D. A. (2018). Transcriptional regulation by Nrf2. Antioxidants & Redox Signaling, 29(17), 1727-1745.

For DNA structure and function:

Alberts, B., Johnson, A., Lewis, J., Morgan, D., Raff, M., Roberts, K., & Walter, P. (2014). Molecular Biology of the Cell (6th ed.). Garland Science.

Watson, J. D., & Crick, F. H. (1953). Molecular structure of nucleic acids. Nature, 171(4356), 737-738.

For epigenetics and its effects:

Weinhold, B. (2006). Epigenetics: the science of change. Environmental Health Perspectives, 114(3), A160-A167.

Feinberg, A. P. (2018). The key role of epigenetics in human disease prevention and mitigation. New England Journal of Medicine, 378(14), 1323-1334.

For exercise-induced epigenetic changes:

Voisin, S., Eynon, N., Yan, X., & Bishop, D. J. (2015). Exercise training and DNA methylation in humans. Acta Physiologica, 213(1), 39-59.

Denham, J., Marques, F. Z., O'Brien, B. J., & Charchar, F. J. (2014). Exercise: putting action into our epigenome. Sports Medicine, 44(2), 189-209

Chapter 5

For the benefits of listening to music while walking:

Karageorghis, C. I., & Priest, D. L. (2012). Music in the exercise domain: a review and synthesis (Part I). InternaƧonal Review of Sport and Exercise Psychology, 5(1), 44-66.

Bigliassi, M., Karageorghis, C. I., Wright, M. J., Orgs, G., & Nowicky, A. V. (2017). Effects of auditory stimuli on electrical activity in the brain during cycle ergometry. Physiology & Behavior, 177, 135-147.

For the benefits of listening to podcasts or audiobooks while walking:

Rebar, A. L., Stanton, R., Geard, D., Short, C., Duncan, M. J., & Vandelanotte, C. (2015). A meta-meta-analysis of the effect of physical activity on depression and anxiety in non-clinical adult populations. Health Psychology Review, 9(3), 366-378.

Flett, J. A., Hayne, H., Riordan, B. C., Thompson, L. M., & Conner, T. S. (2019). Mobile mindfulness meditation: a randomised controlled trial of the effect of two popular apps on mental health. Mindfulness, 10(5), 863-876.

For the benefits of forest walking (shinrin-yoku or forest bathing):

Hansen, M. M., Jones, R., & Tocchini, K. (2017). Shinrin-yoku (forest bathing) and nature therapy: A state-of-the-art review. International Journal of Environmental Research and Public Health, 14(8), 851.

Li, Q. (2010). Effect of forest bathing trips on human immune function. Environmental Health and Preventive Medicine, 15(1), 9-17.

For the effects of phytoncides on human health:

Li, Q., Kobayashi, M., Wakayama, Y., Inagaki, H., Katsumata, M., Hirata, Y., ... & Miyazaki, Y. (2009). Effect of phytoncide from trees on human natural killer cell funcƧon. International Journal of Immunopathology and Pharmacology, 22(4), 951-959.

Ikei, H., Song, C., & Miyazaki, Y. (2017). Physiological effects of wood on humans: a review. Journal of Wood Science, 63(1), 1-23.

For the concept of Directed Attention Fatigue:

Kaplan, S. (1995). The restorative benefits of nature: Toward an integrative framework. Journal of Environmental Psychology, 15(3), 169-182.

Berman, M. G., Jonides, J., & Kaplan, S. (2008). The cognitive benefits of interacƧng with nature. Psychological Science, 19(12), 1207-1212.

For the effects of nature on stress reduction and mood improvement:

Bratman, G. N., Hamilton, J. P., & Daily, G. C. (2012). The impacts of nature experience on human cognitive function and mental health. Annals of the New York Academy of Sciences, 1249(1), 118-136.

Bowler, D. E., Buyung-Ali, L. M., Knight, T. M., & Pullin, A. S. (2010). A systematic review of evidence for the added benefits to health of exposure to natural environments. BMC Public Health, 10(1), 456.

For the benefits of walking meditaɕon:

Prakhinkit, S., Suppapitiporn, S., Tanaka, H., & Suksom, D. (2014). Effects of Buddhism walking meditation on depression, functional fitness, and endothelium-dependent vasodilation in depressed elderly. The Journal of Alternative and Complementary Medicine, 20(5), 411-416.

Teut, M., Roesner, E. J., Ortiz, M., Reese, F., Binting, S., Roll, S., ... & Brinkhaus, B. (2013). Mindful walking in psychologically distressed individuals: A randomized controlled trial. Evidence-Based Complementary and Alternative Medicine, 2013.

Chapter 6

For the discovery and initial studies of Klotho:

Kuro-o, M., Matsumura, Y., Aizawa, H., Kawaguchi, H., Suga, T., Utsugi, T., ... & Nabeshima, Y. I. (1997). Mutaɕon of the mouse klotho gene leads to a syndrome resembling ageing. Nature, 390(6655), 45-51.

Kurosu, H., Yamamoto, M., Clark, J. D., Pastor, J. V., Nandi, A., Gurnani, P., ... & Kuro-o, M. (2005). Suppression of aging in mice by the hormone Klotho. Science, 309(5742), 1829-1833.

For Klotho's role as a myokine and its production in response to exercise:

Safdar, A., & Tarnopolsky, M. A. (2018). Exosomes as mediators of the systemic adaptations to endurance exercise. Cold Spring Harbor Perspectives in Medicine, 8(3), a029827.

Avin, K. G., Coen, P. M., Huang, W., Stolz, D. B., Sowa, G. A., Dubé, J. J., ... & Nederveen, J. P. (2014). Skeletal muscle as a regulator of the longevity protein, Klotho. FronɕGers in Physiology, 5, 189.

For Klotho's anti-aging effects and its role in cognitive funcɕon:

Dubal, D. B., Yokoyama, J. S., Zhu, L., Broestl, L., Worden, K., Wang, D., ... & Mucke, L. (2014). Life extension factor klotho enhances cogniɕon. Cell Reports, 7(4), 1065-1076.

Massó, A., Sánchez, A., Gimenez-Llort, L., Lizcano, J. M., Cañete, M., García, B., ... & Chillon, M. (2015). Secreted and transmembrane Klotho isoforms have different spatio-temporal profiles in the brain during aging and Alzheimer's disease progression. PloS One, 10(11), e0143623.

For Klotho's role in kidney health:

Hu, M. C., Shi, M., Zhang, J., Quiñones, H., Griffith, C., Kuro-o, M., & Moe, O. W. (2011). Klotho deficiency causes vascular calcification in chronic kidney disease. Journal of the American Society of Nephrology, 22(1), 124-136.

Kuro-o, M. (2019). The Klotho proteins in health and disease. Nature Reviews

Nephrology, 15(1), 27-44.

For Klotho's effects on cardiovascular health:

Maltese, G., PseQeli, P. M., Rizzo, B., Srivastava, S., Gnudi, L., Mann, G. E., & Siow, R. C. (2017). The anti-ageing hormone klotho induces Nrf2-mediated anǦoxidant defences in human aortic smooth muscle cells. Journal of Cellular and Molecular Medicine, 21(3), 621-627.

Navarro-González, J. F., Donate-Correa, J., Muros de Fuentes, M., Pérez-Hernández, H., Martinez-Sanz, R., & Mora-Fernández, C. (2014). Reduced Klotho is associated with the presence and severity of coronary artery disease. Heart, 100(1), 34-40.

For Klotho's role in metabolic regulation:

Lin, Y., & Sun, Z. (2015). Antiaging gene Klotho enhances glucose-induced insulin secretion by up-regulating plasma membrane levels of TRPV2 in MIN6 β-cells. Endocrinology, 156(9), 3114-3123.

Yokoyama, J. S., Fukuda, H., Hsieh, C. L., Engelman, C. D., & Dubal, D. B. (2020). Association of the longevity gene KLOTHO with behavioral resilience in older adults. TranslaǦonal Psychiatry, 10(1), 1-9.

For Klotho's association with frailty and mortality:

Shardell, M., Semba, R. D., Rosano, C., Kalyani, R. R., Bandinelli, S., Chia, C. W., & Ferrucci, L. (2019). Plasma klotho and cognitive decline in older adults: findings from the InCHIANTI study. The Journals of Gerontology: Series A, 74(6), 794-800.

Semba, R. D., Cappola, A. R., Sun, K., Bandinelli, S., Dalal, M., Crasto, C., ... & Ferrucci, L. (2011). Plasma klotho and mortality risk in older community-dwelling adults. The Journals of Gerontology: Series A, 66(7), 794-800.

Chapter 7

For diaphragmatic breathing and its benefits:

Ma, X., Yue, Z. Q., Gong, Z. Q., Zhang, H., Duan, N. Y., Shi, Y. T., ... & Li, Y. F. (2017). The effect of diaphragmaǦc breathing on attention, negative affect and stress in healthy adults. Frontiers in Psychology, 8, 874.

Hamasaki, H. (2020). Effects of diaphragmatic breathing on health: a narrative review. Medicines, 7(10), 65.

For pursed-lip breathing:

Cabral, L. F., D'Elia, T. C., Marins, D. S., Zin, W. A., & Guimarães, Γ. S. (2015). Pursed lip breathing improves exercise tolerance in COPD: a randomized crossover study. European Journal of Physical and Rehabilitation Medicine, 51(1), 79-88.

Spahija, J., de Marchie, M., & Grassino, A. (2005). Effects of imposed pursed-lips breathing on respiratory mechanics and dyspnea at rest and during exercise in COPD. Chest, 128(2), 640-650.

For Inspiratory Muscle Strength Training (IMST) and its effects on blood pressure:

Craighead, D. H., Heinbockel, T. C., Hamilton, M. N., Bailey, E. F., MacDonald, M. J., Gibala, M. J., & Seals, D. R. (2021). Time-efficient inspiratory muscle strength training lowers blood pressure and improves endothelial function, NO bioavailability, and oxidative stress in midlife/older adults with above-normal blood pressure. Journal of the American Heart AssociaGon, 10(13), e020980.

DeLucia, C. M., De Asis, R. M., & Bailey, E. F. (2018). Daily inspiratory muscle training lowers blood pressure and vascular resistance in healthy men and women. Experimental Physiology, 103(2), 201-211.

For humming and nitric oxide producGon:

Weitzberg, E., & Lundberg, J. O. (2002). Humming greatly increases nasal nitric oxide. American Journal of Respiratory and Critical Care Medicine, 166(2), 144-145.

Lundberg, J. O., Maniscalco, M., Sofia, M., Lundblad, L., & Weitzberg, E. (2003). Humming, nitric oxide, and paranasal sinus obstruction. JAMA, 289(3), 302-303.

For the importance of nitric oxide in the body:

Förstermann, U., & Sessa, W. C. (2012). Nitric oxide synthases: regulation and funcGon. European Heart Journal, 33(7), 829-837.

Lundberg, J. O., Weitzberg, E., & Gladwin, M. T. (2008). The nitrate–nitrite–nitric oxide pathway in physiology and therapeuGcs. Nature Reviews Drug Discovery, 7(2), 156-167.

For the role of oral bacteria in nitrate-nitrite-NO pathway:

Doel, J. J., Benjamin, N., Hector, M. P., Rogers, M., & Allaker, R. P. (2005). Evaluation of bacterial nitrate reduction in the human oral cavity. European Journal of Oral Sciences, 113(1), 14-19.

Hyde, E. R., Andrade, F., Vaksman, Z., Parthasarathy, K., Jiang, H., Parthasarathy, D. K., ... & Bryan, N. S. (2014). Metagenomic analysis of nitrate-reducing bacteria in the oral cavity: implications for nitric oxide homeostasis. PLoS One, 9(3), e88645.

For the general importance of proper breathing techniques:

Zaccaro, A., Piarulli, A., Laurino, M., Garbella, E., Menicucci, D., Neri, B., & Gemignani, A. (2018). How breath-control can change your life: a systematic review on psycho-physiological correlates of slow breathing. Frontiers in Human Neuroscience, 12, 353.

Russo, M. A., Santarelli, D. M., & O'Rourke, D. (2017). The physiological effects of slow breathing in the healthy human. Breathe, 13(4), 298-309.

Chapter 9

For neurogenesis and BDNF producGon:

Voss, M. W., Vivar, C., Kramer, A. F., & van Praag, H. (2013). Bridging animal and human models of exercise-induced brain plasticity. Trends in Cognitive Sciences, 17(10), 525-544.

Sleiman, S. F., Henry, J., Al-Haddad, R., El Hayek, L., Abou Haidar, E., Stringer, T., ... & Chao, M. V. (2016). Exercise promotes the expression of brain derived neurotrophic factor (BDNF) through the action of the ketone body β-hydroxybutyrate. eLife, 5, e15092.

For reduction of brain cell death:

Belviranlı, M., & Okudan, N. (2018). Exercise training protects against aging-induced cogniGve dysfunction via activation of the hippocampal PGC-1α/FNDC5/BDNF pathway. Neuromolecular Medicine, 20(3), 386-400.

Marosi, K., & Mattson, M. P. (2014). BDNF mediates adaptive brain and body responses to energetic challenges. Trends in Endocrinology & Metabolism, 25(2), 89-98.

For improved mitochondrial funcGon:

Steiner, J. L., Murphy, E. A., McClellan, J. L., Carmichael, M. D., & Davis, J. M. (2011). Exercise training increases mitochondrial biogenesis in the brain. Journal of Applied Physiology, 111(4), 1066-1071.

Marques-Aleixo, I., Oliveira, P. J., Moreira, P. I., Magalhães, J., & Ascensão, A. (2012). Physical exercise as a possible strategy for brain protection: evidence from mitochondrial-mediated mechanisms. Progress in Neurobiology, 99(2), 149-162.

For reduction of oxidative stress:

Radak, Z., Zhao, Z., Koltai, E., Ohno, H., & Atalay, M. (2013). Oxygen consumption and usage during physical exercise: the balance between oxidative stress and ROS-dependent adaptive signaling. Antioxidants & Redox Signaling, 18(10), 1208-1246.

de Sousa, C. V., Sales, M. M., Rosa, T. S., Lewis, J. E., de Andrade, R. V., & Simões, H. G. (2017). The antioxidant effect of exercise: a systematic review and meta-analysis. Sports Medicine, 47(2), 277-293.

For Increased autophagy:

He, C., Sumpter Jr, R., & Levine, B. (2012). Exercise induces autophagy in peripheral tissues and in the brain. Autophagy, 8(10), 1548-1551.

Rocchi, A., & He, C. (2017). Regulation of exercise-induced autophagy in skeletal muscle. Current Pathobiology Reports, 5(2), 177-186.

For reduction of inflammation:

Svensson, M., Lexell, J., & Deierborg, T. (2015). Effects of physical exercise on neuroinflammation, neuroplasticity, neurodegeneration, and behavior: what we can learn from animal models in clinical set t i ngs. Neurorehabilitation and Neural Repair, 29(6), 577-589.

Spielman, L. J., Little, J. P., & Klegeris, A. (2016). Physical activity and exercise attenuate neuroinflammation in neurological diseases. Brain Research Bulletin, 125, 19-29.

For reduced amyloid beta and tau production:

Brown, B. M., Peiffer, J. J., & Martins, R. N. (2013). Multiple effects of physical activity on molecular and cognitive signs of brain aging: can exercise slow neurodegeneration and delay Alzheimer's disease? Molecular Psychiatry, 18(8), 864-874.

Jia, R. X., Liang, J. H., Xu, Y., & Wang, Y. Q. (2019). Effects of physical activity and exercise on the cognitive function of patients with Alzheimer disease: a meta-analysis. BMC Geriatrics, 19(1), 181.

For reducGon in stress hormones:

Heijnen, S., Hommel, B., Kibele, A., & Colzato, L. S. (2016). Neuromodulation of aerobic exercise—a review. Frontiers in Psychology, 6, 1890.

Chen, C., Nakagawa, S., An, Y., Ito, K., Kitaichi, Y., & Kusumi, I. (2017). The exercise-glucocorticoid paradox: How exercise is beneficial for cognition, mood, and the brain while increasing glucocorticoid levels. Frontiers in Neuroendocrinology, 44, 83-102.

For improvement in sleep quality:

Kredlow, M. A., Capozzoli, M. C., Hearon, B. A., Calkins, A. W., & Otto, M. W. (2015). The effects of physical activity on sleep: a meta-analytic review. Journal of Behavioral Medicine, 38(3), 427-449.

Dolezal, B. A., Neufeld, E. V., Boland, D. M., Martin, J. L., & Cooper, C. B. (2017). Interrelationship between sleep and exercise: a systematic review. Advances in Preventive Medicine, 2017.

For improved mood and cognitive function:

Mandolesi, L., Polverino, A., Montuori, S., FoG, F., Ferraioli, G., Sorrentino, P., & Sorrentino, G. (2018). Effects of physical exercise on cognitive functioning and wellbeing: biological and psychological benefits. Frontiers in Psychology, 9, 509.

Basso, J. C., & Suzuki, W. A. (2017). The effects of acute exercise on mood, cognition, neurophysiology, and neurochemical pathways: a review. Brain Plasticity, 2(2), 127-152.

Chapter 11

Discovery of irisin:

Boström, P., Wu, J., Jedrychowski, M. P., Korde, A., Ye, L., Lo, J. C., ... & Spiegelman, B. M. (2012). A PGC1-α-dependent myokine that drives brown-fat-like development of white fat and thermogenesis. Nature, 481(7382), 463-468.

Perakakis, N., Triantafyllou, G. A., Fernández-Real, J. M., Huh, J. Y., Park, K. H., Seufert, J., & Mantzoros, C. S. (2017). Physiology and role of irisin in glucose homeostasis. Nature Reviews Endocrinology, 13(6), 324-337.

Irisin's role in fat browning:

Zhang, Y., Li, R., Meng, Y., Li, S., Donelan, W., Zhao, Y., ... & Tang, D. (2014). Irisin stimulates browning of white adipocytes through mitogen-activated protein kinase p38 MAP kinase and ERK MAP kinase signaling. Diabetes, 63(2), 514-525.

Jeremic, N., Chaturvedi, P., & Tyagi, S. C. (2017). Browning of white fat: novel insight into factors, mechanisms, and therapeutics. Journal of Cellular Physiology, 232(1), 61-68.

Irisin and telomere length:

Rana, K. S., Arif, M., Hill, E. J., Aldred, S., Nagel, D. A., Nevill, A., ... & Brown, J. E. (2014). Plasma irisin levels predict telomere length in healthy adults. Age, 36(2), 995-1001.

Esposito, K., Contaldi, P., Di Mauro, M., Di Pasquale, M., Giugliano, D., & Marfella, R. (2020). Irisin and telomere length in primary prevention of cardiovascular disease. International Journal of Cardiology, 305, 51-55.

Irisin's role in neurogenesis:

Wrann, C. D., White, J. P., Salogiannnis, J., Laznik-Bogoslavski, D., Wu, J., Ma, D., ... & Spiegelman, B. M. (2013). Exercise induces hippocampal BDNF through a PGC-1α/FNDC5 pathway. Cell Metabolism, 18(5), 649-659.

Islam, M. R., Young, M. F., & Wrann, C. D. (2017). The role of FNDC5/Irisin in the nervous system and as a mediator for beneficial effects of exercise on the brain. In Hormones, Metabolism and the Benefits of Exercise (pp. 93-102). Springer, Cham.

Metabolic regulation by irisin:

Huh, J. Y., Panagiotou, G., Mougios, V., Brinkoetter, M., Vamvini, M. T., Schneider, B. E., & Mantzoros, C. S. (2012). FNDC5 and irisin in humans: I. Predictors of circulating concentrations in serum and plasma and II. mRNA expression and circulating concentrations in response to weight loss and exercise. Metabolism, 61(12), 1725-1738.

Xiong, X. Q., Chen, D., Sun, H. J., Ding, L., Wang, J. J., Chen, Q., ... & Zhu, G. Q. (2015). FNDC5 overexpression and irisin ameliorate glucose/lipid metabolic derangements and enhance lipolysis in obesity. Biochimica et Biophysica Acta (BBA)-Molecular Basis of Disease, 1852(9), 1867-1875.

NeuroprotecÇve effects of irisin:

Lourenco, M. V., Frozza, R. L., de Freitas, G. B., Zhang, H., Kincheski, G. C., Ribeiro, F. C., ... & De Felice, F. G. (2019). Exercise-linked FNDC5/irisin rescues synaptic plasticity and memory defects in Alzheimer's models. Nature Medicine, 25(1), 165-175.

Jin, Y., Sumsuzzman, D. M., Choi, J., Kang, H., Lee, S. R., & Hong, Y. (2018). Molecular and functional interaction of the myokine irisin with physical exercise and Alzheimer's disease. Molecules, 23(12), 3229.

Cardiovascular health benefits of irisin:

BaÇrel, S., Bozaykut, P., Mutlu Altundag, E., Kartal Ozer, N., & Mantzoros, C. S. (2014). The effect of irisin on antioxidant system in liver. Free Radical Biology and Medicine, 75, S16.

Chen, J. Q., Huang, Y. Y., Gusdon, A. M., & Qu, S. (2015). Irisin: a new molecular marker and target in metabolic disorder. Lipids in Health and Disease, 14(1), 1-6.

Irisin's acÇvaÇon of SIRT1:

Huh, J. Y., Mougios, V., Kabasakalis, A., Fatouros, I., Siopi, A., Douroudos, I. I., ... & Mantzoros, C. S. (2014). Exercise-induced irisin secretion is independent of age or fitness level and increased irisin may directly modulate muscle metabolism through AMPK activation. The Journal of Clinical Endocrinology & Metabolism, 99(11), E2154-E2161.

Xin, C., Liu, J., Zhang, J., Zhu, D., Wang, H., Xiong, L., ... & Tao, L. (2016). Irisin improves fatty acid oxidation and glucose utilization in type 2 diabetes by regulating the AMPK signaling pathway. International Journal of Obesity, 40(3), 443-451.

Irisin's role in autophagy:

Kim, H., Wrann, C. D., Jedrychowski, M., Vidoni, S., Kitase, Y., Nagano, K., ... & Spiegelman, B. M. (2018). Irisin mediates effects on bone and fat via αV integrin receptors. Cell, 175(7), 1756-1768.

Song, H., Wu, F., Zhang, Y., Zhang, Y., Wang, F., Jiang, M., ... & Li, B. A. (2014). Irisin promotes human umbilical vein endothelial cell proliferation through the ERK signaling pathway and partly suppresses high glucose-induced apoptosis. PloS One, 9(10), e110273.

Irisin's effect on telomerase activation:

Krist, J., Wieder, K., KlöGng, N., Oberbach, A., Kralisch, S., Wiesner, T., ... & Blüher, M. (2013). Effects of weight loss and exercise on apelin serum concentrations and adipose tissue expression in human obesity. Obesity Facts, 6(1), 57-69.

Ost, M., Coleman, V., Kasch, J., & Klaus, S. (2016). Regulation of myokine expression: Role of exercise and cellular stress. Free Radical Biology and Medicine, 98, 78-89.

Chapter 12

History and definition of rucking:

Knapik, J. J., Reynolds, K. L., & Harman, E. (2004). Soldier load carriage: historical, physiological, biomechanical, and medical aspects. Military Medicine, 169(1), 45-56.

Orr, R. M., Pope, R., Johnston, V., & Coyle, J. (2014). Soldier occupational load carriage: a narrative review of associated injuries. International Journal of Injury Control and Safety Promotion, 21(4), 388-396.

Rucking's effects on strength, endurance, and fitness:

Drain, J., Billing, D., Neesham-Smith, D., & Aisbett, B. (2016). Predicting physiological capacity of human load carriage - a review. Applied Ergonomics, 52, 85-94.

Crowder, T. A., Beekley, M. D., Sturdivant, R. X., Johnson, C. A., & Lumpkin, A. (2007). Metabolic effects of soldier performance on a simulated graded road march while wearing two different types of backpacks. Military Medicine, 172(6), 596-602.

Rucking's impact on muscle power and bone health in older adults:

Mori, H., Kuramoto, N., Toi, N., & Nakamura, T. (2020). Effect of a 12-week walking exercise with load on bone metabolism, physical function, and body composition in community-dwelling elderly individuals. Journal of Clinical Medicine, 9(12), 3947.

Conley, K. M., Bice, M. R., Bolin, J. S., & Davis, S. E. (2018). The impact of load carriage on measures of power and agility in tactical occupations: A critical review. International Journal of Environmental Research and Public Health, 15(1), 88.

Calorie expenditure during rucking:

Epstein, Y., Rosenblum, J., Burstein, R., & Sawka, M. N. (1988). External load can alter the energy cost of prolonged exercise. European Journal of Applied Physiology and Occupational Physiology, 57(2), 243-247.

Bastien, G. J., Willems, P. A., Schepens, B., & Heglund, N. C. (2005). Effect of load and speed on the energetic cost of human walking. European Journal of Applied Physiology, 94(1-2), 76-83.

Weight-bearing exercise and bone health:

Kohrt, W. M., Bloomfield, S. A., Little, K. D., Nelson, M. E., & Yingling, V. R. (2004). American College of Sports Medicine Position Stand: physical activity and bone health. Medicine and Science in Sports and Exercise, 36(11), 1985-1996.

Benedeᴎ, M. G., Furlini, G., Zati, A., & Letizia Mauro, G. (2018). The effectiveness of physical exercise on bone density in osteoporotic patients. BioMed Research International, 2018.

Bone deterioration with age:

Khosla, S., & Riggs, B. L. (2005). Pathophysiology of age-related bone loss and osteoporosis. Endocrinology and Metabolism Clinics, 34(4), 1015-1030.

DemonᏅero, O., Vidal, C., & Duque, G. (2012). Aging and bone loss: new insights for the clinician. Therapeuvc Advances in Musculoskeletal Disease, 4(2), 61-76.

Exercise and bone health in aging:

Gómez-Cabello, A., Ara, I., González-Agüero, A., Casajús, J. A., & Vicente-Rodríguez, G. (2012). Effects of training on bone mass in older adults. Sports Medicine, 42(4), 301-325.

Bolam, K. A., Van Uffelen, J. G., & Taaffe, D. R. (2013). The effect of physical exercise on bone density in middle-aged and older men: a systematic review. Osteoporosis International, 24(11), 2749-2762.

Chapter 14

1. S. Moncada, E.A. Higgs, The discovery of nitric oxide and its role in vascular biology, British Journal of Pharmacology (2006) 147, S193–S201.

2. Vanhoutte PM, Shimokawa H, Tang EH, Feletou M. Endothelial dysfunction and vascular disease. Acta Physiol (Oxf). 2009 Jun;196(2):193-222.

3. Radomski MW, Palmer RM, Moncada S. An L-arginine/nitric oxide pathway present in human platelets regulates aggregation. Proc Natl Acad Sci U S A. 1990 Jul;87(13):5193-7.

4. Garthwaite J. Concepts of neural nitric oxide-mediated transmission. Eur J Neurosci. 2008 Jun;27(11):2783-802.

5. Calabrese V, Mancuso C, Calvani M, Rizzarelli E, Butterfield DA, Stella AM. Nitric oxide in the central nervous system: neuroprotection versus neurotoxicity. Nat Rev Neurosci. 2007 Oct;8(10):766-75.

6. Hervera A, et al. Reactive oxygen species regulate axonal regeneration through the release of exosomal NADPH oxidase 2 complexes into injured axons. Nat Cell Biol. 2018 Mar;20(3):307-319.

7. Bogdan C. Nitric oxide synthase in innate and adaptive immunity: an update. Trends Immunol. 2015 Mar;36(3):161-78.

8. Bettelli E, et al. Reciprocal developmental pathways for the generation of pathogenic effector TH17 and regulatory T cells. Nature. 2006 May 11;441(7090):235-8.

9. Bloor CM. Angiogenesis during exercise and training. Angiogenesis. 2005;8(3):263-71.

10. Bradley EA, et al. Meşormin improves vascular and metabolic insulin action in insulin-resistant muscle. J Endocrinol. 2019 Nov;243(2):85-96.

11. Guzik TJ, Korbut R, Adamek-Guzik T. Nitric oxide and superoxide in inflammation and immune regulaҫion. J Physiol Pharmacol. 2003 Dec;54(4):469-87.

Chapter 15

Information Theory of Aging:

Sinclair, D. A., & LaPlante, M. D. (2019). Lifespan: Why we age—and why we don't have to. Atria Books.

López-Orn, C., Blasco, M. A., Partridge, L., Serrano, M., & Kroemer, G. (2013). The hallmarks of aging. Cell, 153(6), 1194-1217.

Longevity Genes (Sirtuins, mTOR, AMPK):

Bonkowski, M. S., & Sinclair, D. A. (2016). Slowing ageing by design: the rise of NAD+ and sirtuin-activating compounds. Nature Reviews Molecular Cell Biology, 17(11), 679-690.

Weichhart, T. (2018). mTOR as regulator of lifespan, aging, and cellular senescence: a mini-review. Gerontology, 64(2), 127-134.

Cellular Reprogramming:

Ocampo, A., Reddy, P., Marҫnez-Redondo, P., Platero-Luengo, A., Hatanaka, F., Hishida, T., ... & Izpisua Belmonte, J. C. (2016). In vivo amelioration of age-associated hallmarks by partial reprogramming. Cell, 167(7), 1719-1733.

Lu, Y., Brommer, B., Tian, X., Krishnan, A., Meer, M., Wang, C., ... & Sinclair, D. A. (2020). Reprogramming to recover youthful epigenetic information and restore vision. Nature, 588(7836), 124-129.

Lifestyle Interventions (Intermittent Fasting, Exercise):

de Cabo, R., & Mattson, M. P. (2019). Effects of intermittent fasting on health, aging, and disease. New England Journal of Medicine, 381(26), 2541-2551.

Garatachea, N., Pareja-Galeano, H., Sanchis-Gomar, F., Santos-Lozano, A., Fiuza-Luces, C., Morán, M., ... & Lucia, A. (2015). Exercise attenuates the major hallmarks of aging. Rejuvenation Research, 18(1), 57-89.

Potential Longevity Molecules (Resveratrol, NAD+ boosters, Metformin, Rapamycin):

Blagosklonny, M. V. (2019). Rapamycin for longevity: opinion article. Aging (Albany NY), 11(19), 8048.

Balasubramanian, P., Howell, P. R., & Anderson, R. M. (2017). Aging and caloric restriction research: a biological perspective with translational potential. EBioMedicine, 21, 37-44.

Ethical and Societal Implications of Life Extension:

Partridge, B., Lucke, J., Bartlett, H., & Hall, W. (2009). Ethical, social, and personal implications of extended human lifespan identified by members of the public. Rejuvenation Research, 12(5), 351-357.

Gems, D. (2015). The aging-disease false dichotomy: understanding senescence as pathology. Frontiers in Genetics, 6, 212.

Future of Longevity Research:

Kennedy, B. K., Berger, S. L., Brunet, A., Campisi, J., Cuervo, A. M., Epel, E. S., ... & Sierra, F. (2014). Geroscience: linking aging to chronic disease. Cell, 159(4), 709-713.

Barzilai, N., Crandall, J. P., Kritchevsky, S. B., & Espeland, M. A. (2016). Metformin as a tool to target aging. Cell Metabolism, 23(6), 1060-1065.

Chapter 16

AMPK structure and activation:

Hardie, D. G., Ross, F. A., & Hawley, S. A. (2012). AMPK: a nutrient and energy sensor that maintains energy homeostasis. Nature Reviews Molecular Cell Biology, 13(4), 251-262.

Herzig, S., & Shaw, R. J. (2018). AMPK: guardian of metabolism and mitochondrial homeostasis. Nature Reviews Molecular Cell Biology, 19(2), 121-135.

AMPK's role in glucose metabolism:

Viollet, B., Horman, S., Leclerc, J., LanGer, L., Foretz, M., Billaud, M., ... & Andreelli, F. (2010). AMPK inhibition in health and disease. Critical Reviews in Biochemistry and Molecular Biology, 45(4), 276-295.

Jeon, S. M. (2016). RegulaGon and function of AMPK in physiology and diseases. Experimental & Molecular Medicine, 48(7), e245-e245.

AMPK's role in lipid metabolism:

Fullerton, M. D. (2016). AMP-activated protein kinase and its mulGfaceted regulaGon of hepaGc metabolism. Current Opinion in Lipidology, 27(2), 172-180.

Day, E. A., Ford, R. J., & Steinberg, G. R. (2017). AMPK as a therapeutic target for treating metabolic diseases. Trends in Endocrinology & Metabolism, 28(8), 545-560.

AMPK and autophagy:

Kim, J., Kundu, M., Viollet, B., & Guan, K. L. (2011). AMPK and mTOR regulate autophagy through direct phosphorylation of Ulk1. Nature Cell Biology, 13(2), 132-141.

Mihaylova, M. M., & Shaw, R. J. (2011). The AMPK signalling pathway coordinates cell growth, autophagy and metabolism. Nature Cell Biology, 13(9), 1016-1023.

AMPK and mitochondrial biogenesis:

Fernandez-Marcos, P. J., & Auwerx, J. (2011). Regulation of PGC-1α, a nodal regulator of mitochondrial biogenesis. The American Journal of Clinical Nutrition, 93(4), 884S-890S.

Cantó, C., & Auwerx, J. (2009). PGC-1alpha, SIRT1 and AMPK, an energy sensing network that controls energy expenditure. Current Opinion in Lipidology, 20(2), 98-105.

AMPK and aging:

Salminen, A., & Kaarniranta, K. (2012). AMP-activated protein kinase (AMPK) controls the aging process via an integrated signaling network. Ageing Research Reviews, 11(2), 230-241.

Burkewitz, K., Zhang, Y., & Mair, W. B. (2014). AMPK at the nexus of energetics and aging. Cell Metabolism, 20(1), 10-25.

AMPK and exercise:

Kjøbsted, R., Hingst, J. R., Fentz, J., Foretz, M., Sanz, M. N., Pehmøller, C., ... & Wojtaszewski, J. F. (2018). AMPK in skeletal muscle functivon and metabolism. The FASEB Journal, 32(4), 1741-1777.

Richter, E. A., & Ruderman, N. B. (2009). AMPK and the biochemistry of exercise: implications for human health and disease. Biochemical Journal, 418(2), 261-275.

AMPK and insulin signaling:

Friedrichsen, M., Mortensen, B., Pehmøller, C., Birk, J. B., & Wojtaszewski, J. F. (2013). Exercise-induced AMPK activity in skeletal muscle: role in glucose uptake and insulin sensitivity. Molecular and Cellular Endocrinology, 366(2), 204-214.

Jeon, S. M. (2016). Regulation and function of AMPK in physiology and diseases. Experimental & Molecular Medicine, 48(7), e245-e245.

AMPK and mTOR:

González, A., Hall, M. N., Lin, S. C., & Hardie, D. G. (2020). AMPK and TOR: The Yin and Yang of Cellular Nutrient Sensing and Growth Control. Cell Metabolism, 31(3), 472-492.

Saxton, R. A., & Sabaǥni, D. M. (2017). mTOR signaling in growth, metabolism, and disease. Cell, 168(6), 960-976.

AMPK and sirtuins:

Cantó, C., & Auwerx, J. (2009). PGC-1alpha, SIRT1 and AMPK, an energy sensing network that controls energy expenditure. Current Opinion in Lipidology, 20(2), 98-105.

Ruderman, N. B., Xu, X. J., Nelson, L., Cacicedo, J. M., Saha, A. K., Lan, F., & Ido, Y. (2010). AMPK and SIRT1: a long-standing partnership? American Journal of Physiology-Endocrinology and Metabolism, 298(4), E751-E760.

Chapter 17

Resting Heart Rate (RHR):

Aune, D., Sen, A., O'Hartaigh, B., Janszky, I., Romundstad, P. R., Tonstad, S., & Vatten, L. J. (2017). Resting heart rate and the risk of cardiovascular disease, total cancer, and all-cause mortality—A systematic review and dose—response meta-analysis of prospective studies. Nutrition, Metabolism and Cardiovascular Diseases, 27(6), 504-517.

Jensen, M. T., Suadicani, P., Hein, H. O., & Gyntelberg, F. (2013). Elevated resting heart rate, physical fitness and all-cause mortality: a 16-year follow-up in the Copenhagen Male Study. Heart, 99(12), 882-887.

Body Mass Index (BMI):

Global BMI Mortality Collaboration. (2016). Body-mass index and all-cause mortality: individual-participant-data meta-analysis of 239 prospective studies. The Lancet, 388(10046), 776-786.

Bhaskaran, K., Dos-Santos-Silva, I., Leon, D. A., Douglas, I. J., & Smeeth, L. (2018). Association of BMI with overall and cause-specific mortality: a population-based cohort study of 3· 6 million adults in the UK. The Lancet Diabetes & Endocrinology, 6(12), 944-953.

Maximal Oxygen ConsumpGon (VO2 max):

Ross, R., Blair, S. N., Arena, R., Church, T. S., Després, J. P., Franklin, B. A., ... & Wisløff, U. (2016). Importance of assessing cardiorespiratory fitness in clinical practice: a case for fitness as a clinical vital sign: a scientific statement from the American Heart Association. Circulation, 134(24), e653-e699.

Harber, M. P., Kaminsky, L. A., Arena, R., Blair, S. N., Franklin, B. A., Myers, J., & Ross, R. (2017). Impact of cardiorespiratory fitness on all-cause and disease-specific mortality: advances since 2009. Progress in Cardiovascular Diseases, 60(1), 11-20.

Maximum Heart Rate (MHR):

Nes, B. M., Janszky, I., Wisløff, U., Støylen, A., & Karlsen, T. (2013). Age-predicted maximal heart rate in healthy subjects: The HUNT Fitness Study. Scandinavian Journal of Medicine & Science in Sports, 23(6), 697-704.

Gellish, R. L., Goslin, B. R., Olson, R. E., McDonald, A., Russi, G. D., & Moudgil, V. K. (2007). Longitudinal modeling of the relationship between age and maximal heart rate. Medicine and Science in Sports and Exercise, 39(5), 822-829.

Heart Rate Recovery (HRR):

Qiu, S., Cai, X., Sun, Z., Li, L., Zuegel, M., Steinacker, J. M., & Schumann, U. (2017). Heart rate recovery and risk of cardiovascular events and all-cause mortality: a meta-analysis of prospective cohort studies. Journal of the American Heart Association, 6(5), e005505.

Cole, C. R., Blackstone, E. H., Pashkow, F. J., Snader, C. E., & Lauer, M. S. (1999). Heart-rate recovery immediately after exercise as a predictor of mortality. New England Journal of Medicine, 341(18), 1351-1357.

Waist-to-Hip Ratio (WHR):

Seidell, J. C. (2010). Waist circumference and waist/hip ratio in relation to all-cause mortality, cancer and sleep apnea. European Journal of Clinical NutriGon, 64(1), 35-41.

Czernichow, S., Kengne, A. P., Stamatakis, E., Hamer, M., & Batty, G. D. (2011). Body mass index, waist circumference and waist–hip ratio: which is the better discriminator of cardiovascular disease mortality risk? Evidence from an individual-participant meta-analysis of 82 864 participants from nine cohort studies. Obesity Reviews, 12(9), 680-687.

Blood Pressure:

Ettehad, D., Emdin, C. A., Kiran, A., Anderson, S. G., Callender, T., Emberson, J.,

... & Rahimi, K. (2016). Blood pressure lowering for prevention of cardiovascular disease and death: a systematic review and meta-analysis. The Lancet, 387(10022), 957-967.

Whelton, P. K., Carey, R. M., Aronow, W. S., Casey, D. E., Collins, K. J., Himmelfarb, C. D., ... & Wright, J. T. (2018). 2017 ACC/AHA/AAPA/ABC/ACPM/AGS/APhA/ASH/ASPC/NMA/PCNA guideline for the prevention, detection, evaluation, and management of high blood pressure in adults: a report of the American College of Cardiology/American Heart Association Task Force on Clinical Practice Guidelines. Journal of the American College of Cardiology, 71(19), e127-e248.

C-reactive Protein (CRP):

Emerging Risk Factors Collaboration. (2010). C-reactive protein concentration and risk of coronary heart disease, stroke, and mortality: an individual participant meta-analysis. The Lancet, 375(9709), 132-140.

Ridker, P. M. (2016). A test in context: high-sensitivity C-reactive protein. Journal of the American College of Cardiology, 67(6), 712-723.

Basal Metabolic Rate (BMR):

Müller, M. J., Geisler, C., Hübers, M., Pourhassan, M., Braun, W., & Bosy-Westphal, A. (2018). Normalizing resting energy expenditure across the life course in humans: challenges and hopes. European Journal of Clinical Nutriĝon, 72(5), 628-637.

McMurray, R. G., Soares, J., Caspersen, C. J., & McCurdy, T. (2014). Examining variations of resting metabolic rate of adults: a public health perspective. Medicine and Science in Sports and Exercise, 46(7), 1352-1358.

Heart Rate Variability (HRV):

Shaffer, F., & Ginsberg, J. P. (2017). An overview of heart rate variability metrics and norms. Frontiers in Public Health, 5, 258.

Thayer, J. F., Yamamoto, S. S., & Brosschot, J. F. (2010). The relationship of autonomic imbalance, heart rate variability and cardiovascular disease risk factors. Internatitional Journal of Cardiology, 141(2), 122-131.

Blood Glucose Levels (BGL):

American Diabetes Associaĝon. (2020). 2. Classification and diagnosis of diabetes: standards of medical care in diabetes—2020. Diabetes Care, 43(Supplement 1), S14-S31.

Emerging Risk Factors Collaboration. (2010). Diabetes mellitus, fasting blood glucose concentration, and risk of vascular disease: a collaborative meta-analysis of 102 prospective studies. The Lancet, 375(9733), 2215-2222.

Oxygen Saturation (SpO2):

Jubran, A. (2015). Pulse oximetry. Critical Care, 19(1), 272.

Wilson, B. J., Cowan, H. J., Lord, J. A., Zuege, D. J., & Zygun, D. A. (2010). The accuracy of pulse oximetry in emergency department patients with severe sepsis and septic shock: a retrospective cohort study. BMC Emergency Medicine, 10(1), 9.

Glycated Hemoglobin (HbA1c):

American Diabetes Association. (2020). 6. Glycemic targets: standards of medical care in diabetes—2020. Diabetes Care, 43(Supplement 1), S66-S76.

Sherwani, S. I., Khan, H. A., Ekhzaimy, A., Masood, A., & Sakharkar, M. K. (2016). Significance of HbA1c test in diagnosis and prognosis of diabetic patients. Biomarker Insights, 11, BMI-S38440.

Total Cholesterol (TC):

Ference, B. A., Ginsberg, H. N., Graham, I., Ray, K. K., Packard, C. J., Bruckert, E., ... & Catapano, A. L. (2017). Low-density lipoproteins cause atherosclerotic cardiovascular disease. 1. Evidence from genetic, epidemiologic, and clinical studies. A consensus statement from the European Atherosclerosis Society Consensus Panel. European Heart Journal, 38(32), 2459-2472.

Grundy, S. M., Stone, N. J., Bailey, A. L., Beam, C., Birtcher, K. K., Blumenthal, R. S., ... & Yeboah, J. (2019). 2018 AHA/ACC/AACVPR/AAPA/ABC/ACPM/ADA/ AGS/APhA/ASPC/NLA/PCNA guideline on the management of blood cholesterol: a report of the American College of Cardiology/American Heart Association Task Force on Clinical Practice Guidelines. Circulation, 139(25), e1082-e1143.

Low Density Lipoprotein (LDL):

Ference, B. A., Ginsberg, H. N., Graham, I., Ray, K. K., Packard, C. J., Bruckert, E., ... & Catapano, A. L. (2017). Low-density lipoproteins cause atherosclerotic cardiovascular disease. 1. Evidence from genetic, epidemiologic, and clinical studies. A consensus statement from the European Atherosclerosis Society Consensus Panel. European Heart Journal, 38(32), 2459-2472.

Sacks, F. M., Lichtenstein, A. H., Wu, J. H., Appel, L. J., Creager, M. A., Kris-Etherton, P. M., ... & Horn, L. V. (2017). Dietary fats and cardiovascular disease: a presidential advisory from the American Heart Association. Circulation, 136(3), e1-e23.

High Density Lipoprotein (HDL):

Madsen, C. M., Varbo, A., & Nordestgaard, B. G. (2017). Extreme high high-density lipoprotein cholesterol is paradoxically associated with high mortality in men and women: two prospective cohort studies. European Heart Journal, 38(32), 2478-2486.

Rader, D. J., & Hovingh, G. K. (2014). HDL and cardiovascular disease. The Lancet, 384(9943), 618-625.

RECOMMENDED BOOKS

Books on longevity:

1. *Lifespan: Why We Age - and Why We Don't Have To* by David A. Sinclair, PhD (Atria Books, 2019) This groundbreaking book by a leading Harvard researcher presents aging as a treatable disease rather than an inevitable process. Sinclair explains cutting-edge research on aging and presents practical strategies for extending healthspan through genetic and lifestyle interventions.

2. *The Blue Zones* by Dan Buettner (National Geographic Society, 2008) Buettner explores five regions in the world where people live extraordinarily long and healthy lives. Through his research, he identifies common lifestyle factors that contribute to longevity and provides actionable strategies for implementing these principles.

3. *Why We Sleep: Unlocking the Power of Sleep and Dreams* by Matthew Walker (Scribner, 2017) While not exclusively about longevity, this book makes a compelling case for sleep as a crucial factor in health and longevity. Walker, a neuroscientist, explains how quality sleep affects every aspect of our physical and mental health, and how it can extend both lifespan and healthspan.

4. *The Longevity Diet* by Valter Longo, PhD (Avery, 2018) Longo, a leading researcher in longevity, presents his scientifically backed approach to eating for a longer, healthier life. The book combines insights from centenarian populations with cutting-edge research on fasting and dietary interventions for longevity.

5. *Metabolic Autophagy* by Siim Land (Self-published, 2019) This book dives deep into the science of autophagy, the cellular cleanup process crucial for longevity. Land explains complex biological processes in accessible terms and provides practical strategies for activating autophagy through diet and lifestyle.

6. *Growing Young: How Friendship, Optimism, and Kindness Can Help You Live to 100* by Marta Zaraska (Appetite, 2020) Zaraska explores the often-overlooked social and psychological factors that contribute to longevity. She presents compelling research showing how positive relationships and mental outlook can be as important for longevity as diet and exercise.

7. **The Telomere Effect** by Dr. Elizabeth Blackburn and Dr. Elissa Epel (Grand Central Publishing, 2017) Written by a Nobel Prize winner, this book explains how telomeres affect aging and how we can protect them. The authors provide scientific insights and practical recommendations for maintaining telomere health through lifestyle choices.

8. **Super Human** by Dave Asprey (Harper Wave, 2019) Asprey combines traditional wisdom with cutting-edge research to present a comprehensive guide to extending lifespan. The book offers a systematic approach to optimizing biological functions for longevity through various biohacking techniques.

9 **Aging Backwards** by Miranda Esmonde-White (Harper Wave, 2018) This book focuses on the role of movement and exercise in maintaining youth and vitality as we age. Esmonde-White presents a science-based approach to maintaining mobility and preventing age-related physical decline through specific movement patterns.

Books on diet and nutrition:

1. **How Not to Die** by Michael Greger, MD (Flatiron Books, 2015) Dr. Greger examines the leading causes of death and explains how dietary changes can prevent and reverse disease. Based on extensive scientific research, he provides practical dietary recommendations and explains the scientific evidence behind plant-based eating for optimal health.

2. **Deep Nutrition** by Catherine Shanahan, MD (Flatiron Books, 2017) Dr. Shanahan combines anthropological research of traditional diets with modern nutritional science to explain how food affects our genes and health. She presents four key nutritional strategies based on the dietary wisdom of global cultures and explains how modern food processing has disrupted these traditional patterns.

3. **The Omnivore's Dilemma** by Michael Pollan (Penguin Press, 2006) Pollan investigates where our food comes from and the implications of different food production systems on our health and environment. Through four meals from different food chains (industrial, organic, local, and foraged), he illuminates the complex relationships between food, health, and sustainability.

4. **Intuitive Eating** by Evelyn Tribole and Elyse Resch (St. Martin's Essentials, 4th Edition, 2020) This groundbreaking book challenges

traditional dieting approaches and presents a framework for developing a healthy relationship with food. The authors provide practical strategies for reconnecting with hunger and fullness cues while breaking free from the diet mentality.

5. ***Metabolic Effects of Food*** by David Ludwig, MD, PhD (Avid Reader Press, 2021) Dr. Ludwig explains how different foods affect our metabolism, hormones, and weight regulation systems. He presents a science-based approach to nutrition that focuses on food quality rather than just calories, explaining how certain foods can help regulate hunger and metabolism.

6. ***Eat to Beat Disease*** by William Li, MD (Grand Central Publishing, 2019) Dr. Li explains how specific foods can activate the body's health defense systems to fight disease and promote healing. He provides a comprehensive guide to foods that support the body's five defense systems: angiogenesis, cell regeneration, microbiome, DNA protection, and immunity.

7. ***The Blue Zones Kitchen*** by Dan Buettner (National Geographic, 2019) Buettner collects recipes and cooking lessons from the world's longest-lived populations. The book combines fascinating anthropological insights with practical cooking advice, showing how traditional dietary patterns support longevity and health.

8. ***Genius Foods*** by Max Lugavere (Harper Wave, 2018) Lugavere examines the connection between diet and brain health, explaining how specific foods can enhance cognitive function and protect against neurological decline. He presents a comprehensive plan for optimizing brain health through diet, combining cutting-edge research with practical dietary recommendations.

9. ***"The Perfect Health Diet"*** by Paul Jaminet, PhD and Shou-Ching Jaminet, PhD (Scribner, 2012) The authors present a scientifically-based approach to optimal nutrition, drawing from both evolutionary biology and modern research. They explain how to optimize macronutrient ratios and select the most nutritious foods while avoiding common dietary pitfalls.

10. **"Food Rules"** by Michael Pollan (Penguin Books, 2009) Pollan distills complex nutrition science into simple, memorable guidelines for healthy eating. His concise, witty approach makes nutrition accessible to everyone, offering practical wisdom that cuts through the confusion of conflicting dietary advice.

Books on exercise:

1. *Younger Next Year: The Exercise Program* by Chris Crowley and Henry S. Lodge, MD (Workman Publishing, 2015) This book combines cutting-edge science with practical exercise advice specifically tailored for older adults. The authors explain why exercise becomes increasingly crucial as we age and provide detailed workout programs that combine aerobic exercise, strength training, and core work.

2. *Strength Training Past 50* by Wayne Westcott and Thomas Baechle (Human Kinetics, 3rd Edition, 2019) The authors present research-based strength training programs specifically designed for older adults, including modifications for various fitness levels and health conditions. The book includes detailed exercises with clear instructions and photos, focusing on safe and effective techniques for building strength and maintaining muscle mass.

3. *Fitness After 50* by Walter Bortz II, MD (Basic Health Publications, 2015) Dr. Bortz, a longevity expert, explains how exercise can reverse aging effects and maintain functionality throughout life. He provides practical exercise programs that emphasize flexibility, balance, strength, and endurance, with modifications for different fitness levels and health conditions.

4. *Fast After 50* by Joe Friel (VeloPress, 2015) While focused on endurance athletes, this book provides valuable insights for any aging adult interested in maintaining or improving their fitness. Friel explains the physiological changes that occur with aging and provides strategies for adapting training to maintain performance and health.

5. *Dynamic Aging: Simple Exercises for Whole-Body Mobility* by Katy Bowman (Propriometrics Press, 2017) Biomechanist Katy Bowman presents a comprehensive approach to maintaining mobility and functionality through natural movement. The book includes simple, practical exercises that can be integrated into daily life, focusing on maintaining joint mobility and preventing common age-related movement limitations.

6. *Ageless Intensity* by Pete McCall (Human Kinetics, 2021) McCall provides a science-based approach to high-intensity training for older adults, explaining how to safely incorporate more challenging workouts. The book includes detailed workout plans and modifications, emphasizing the importance of recovery and proper progression.

7. *The New Rules of Lifting for Life* by Lou Schuler and Alwyn Cosgrove (Avery, 2012) This comprehensive guide provides adaptable strength training programs that can be modified for any fitness level or physical limitation. The authors emphasize functional movements that support daily activities and include detailed progressions and regressions for each exercise.

8. *Stretching for 50+* by Karl Knopf (Ulysses Press, 2017) Dr. Knopf presents a comprehensive guide to maintaining flexibility and mobility as we age. The book includes detailed stretching routines for different body parts and activities, with modifications for various physical limitations and clear photos demonstrating proper technique.

9. *Brain Rules for Aging Well* by John Medina (Pear Press, 2017) While not exclusively about exercise, this book includes crucial information about how physical activity affects brain health and cognitive function as we age. Medina combines scientific research with practical exercise recommendations for maintaining both physical and mental fitness.

10. *Water Exercise* by Martha White (Human Kinetics, 2017) This book focuses on the benefits of water-based exercise for older adults, providing low-impact workouts that build strength, flexibility, and cardiovascular fitness. The author includes detailed exercise descriptions and workout plans suitable for various fitness levels and physical limitations.

Books on brain health

1. *The Brain That Changes Itself* by Norman Doidge, MD (Penguin Books, 2007) Dr. Doidge explores neuroplasticity, demonstrating how the brain can reorganize and heal itself through specific interventions and exercises. Through compelling case studies and scientific research, he shows how understanding brain plasticity can help overcome various neurological challenges and enhance cognitive function.

2. *Brain Rules* by John Medina (Pear Press, 2014) Medina presents twelve fundamental principles about how the brain works, backed by scientific research and practical applications. He explains complex neuroscience in an accessible way, offering strategies for improving memory, enhancing learning, and optimizing brain performance in daily life.

3. *Keep Sharp: Build a Better Brain at Any Age* by Sanjay Gupta, MD (Simon & Schuster, 2021) Dr. Gupta combines cutting-edge research with practical advice to create a comprehensive plan for maintaining cognitive health throughout life. The book debunks common myths about aging and memory while providing a concrete five-step program for enhancing brain function.

4. *The End of Alzheimer's* by Dale Bredesen, MD (Avery, 2017) Dr. Bredesen presents his revolutionary protocol for preventing and reversing cognitive decline through a comprehensive, personalized approach. He explains the multiple causes of Alzheimer's disease and provides detailed strategies for addressing each through lifestyle modifications, nutritional interventions, and targeted therapies.

5. *Spark: The Revolutionary New Science of Exercise and the Brain* by John J. Ratey, MD (Little, Brown and Company, 2008) Dr. Ratey presents compelling evidence for exercise as a powerful tool for improving brain function and mental health. He explains how physical activity enhances learning, reduces stress and anxiety, fights depression, and sharpens memory.

6. *The Hidden Brain* by Shankar Vedantam (Spiegel & Grau, 2010) Vedantam explores how unconscious biases and mental processes influence our behavior and decision-making. Through fascinating stories and research, he reveals how understanding our hidden brain can help us make better decisions and improve our cognitive function.

7. *Brain Food: The Surprising Science of Eating for Cognitive Power* by Lisa Mosconi, PhD (Avery, 2018) Dr. Mosconi combines neuroscience and nutrition to explain how diet affects brain health and cognitive function. She provides detailed dietary recommendations based on cutting-edge research, explaining which foods best support brain health and why.

8. *TheAge-Proof Brain: New Strategies to Improve Memory, Protect Immunity, and Fight Off Dementia* by Marc Milstein (BenBella Books, 2017) Dr. Milstein makes cutting-edge neuroscience accessible to everyone in this vital guidebook highlighting the critical lifestyle factors that empower you to maintain a sharp, healthy, active brain and protect against dementia.

9. *Changing Mind: Our Brain, Our Potential to Transform Ourselves* by Dr. Daniel J. Siegel (Bantam, 2020) Dr. Siegel explores how understanding the brain's functioning can lead to personal transformation and enhanced mental well-being. He combines neuroscience with mindfulness practices to provide practical strategies for improving focus, emotional regulation, and overall brain health.

10. *The Brain's Way of Healing* by Norman Doidge, MD (Penguin Books, 2016) This follow-up to "The Brain That Changes Itself" explores natural methods for harnessing neuroplasticity to promote healing and enhance brain function. Through remarkable case studies, Dr. Doidge demonstrates how various non-invasive techniques can activate the brain's own healing mechanisms.

Books on walking:

1. *Born to Walk: The Transformative Power of a Simple Act* by Dan Rubinstein (ECW Press, 2015) Rubinstein explores how walking affects our minds, bodies, and societies through research and real-world examples. He demonstrates how this basic human activity can transform physical health, mental well-being, and social connections while offering practical guidance for incorporating more walking into daily life.

2. *In Praise of Walking: A New Scientific Exploration* by Shane O'Mara (W. W. Norton & Company, 2020) A neuroscientist examines walking's profound benefits for our bodies, minds, and emotions through a scientific lens. O'Mara explains how walking makes us smarter, happier, and healthier while sharing compelling research about walking's impact on brain function and overall well-being.

3. *Walking: The Complete Book* by Jeff Galloway (Meyer & Meyer Sport, 2016) Olympic runner Jeff Galloway provides comprehensive guidance for using walking as a primary form of exercise, including training programs for various fitness levels. He offers detailed advice on technique, injury prevention, and goal-setting while explaining how to maximize walking's health benefits.

4. *Chi Walking: Fitness Walking for Lifelong Health and Energy* by Danny Dreyer (Simon & Schuster, 2006) Dreyer combines principles from Tai Chi with walking to create a mindful, energizing approach to fitness walking. The book provides detailed instruction on proper form, breathing techniques, and mental focus to make walking more effective and enjoyable.

5. *The Joy of Walking: Selected Writings* by Suzy Cripps (Notting Hill Editions, 2019) This collection combines scientific insights about walking's benefits with inspiring essays about the pleasure of walking. Cripps explores both the physical and psychological benefits of walking while encouraging readers to develop their own walking practice.

6. *Walking Your Way to Better Health* by Dr. Mark Fenton (Lyons Press, 2018) Dr. Fenton provides evidence-based strategies for using walking to improve health, manage weight, and prevent chronic disease. The book includes detailed walking programs, technique instruction, and guidance for overcoming common obstacles to regular walking.

7. *Nordic Walking: The Complete Guide to Health, Fitness, and Fun* by Claire Walter (Hatherleigh Press, 2009) Walter introduces Nordic walking, explaining how using poles can enhance the benefits of regular walking by engaging more muscle groups. She provides comprehensive instruction on technique, equipment selection, and training programs while explaining the unique advantages of this walking style.

8. *Walking for Health and Happiness: The 30-Day Plan* by William Bird, MD (Reader's Digest, 2014) Dr. Bird presents a structured approach to developing a sustainable walking habit through a 30-day program. He combines medical expertise with practical advice, explaining how to progress safely while maximizing physical and mental health benefits.

9. *Walk Your Way to Better: 99 Walks That Will Change Your Life* by Joyce Shulman (Bound Book Media, 2020) Shulman provides themed walks designed to enhance creativity, reduce stress, and improve problem-solving abilities. Each walk includes specific mindfulness exercises and prompts to make walking a more purposeful and transformative experience.

10. *The First Steps: Understanding Your Walking Journey* by Carolyn Scott Kortge (Meyer & Meyer Sport, 2015) Kortge combines practical walking advice with strategies for overcoming mental barriers to regular exercise. She provides guidance for beginners while addressing common concerns and offering solutions for staying motivated.

Books that explain human physiology in accessible terms:

1. *The Body: A Guide for Occupants* by Bill Bryson (Doubleday, 2019) Bryson takes readers on a head-to-toe tour of the human body,

explaining complex physiological processes with his characteristic wit and clarity. He combines fascinating facts with engaging storytelling to make human anatomy and physiology accessible to anyone, covering everything from the brain to the immune system while weaving in historical discoveries and current research.

2. *Your Body: The Missing Manual* by Matthew MacDonald (O'Reilly Media, 2009) Written like a user's guide for your body, this book explains how all your biological systems work and interact in clear, everyday language. MacDonald demystifies complex bodily processes with helpful analogies, practical examples, and useful tips for optimizing your body's performance.

3. *The Story of the Human Body: Evolution, Health, and Disease* by Daniel Lieberman (Pantheon Books, 2013) Lieberman explains how our bodies evolved and how modern life affects our biological systems, using clear language and relatable examples. He connects evolutionary biology to everyday physiology, helping readers understand why our bodies function the way they do and how modern lifestyle choices impact our health.

4. *How the Body Works: The Facts Simply Explained* (DK Publishing, 2016) This visually rich guide uses clear illustrations and straightforward explanations to demystify human physiology. The book breaks down complex processes into digestible chunks, using infographics and diagrams to explain everything from cellular function to organ systems.

5. *The Human Body Book: An Illustrated Guide to its Structure, Function, and Disorders* by Steve Parker (DK Adult, 2019) This comprehensive reference uses stunning 3D illustrations and clear explanations to make anatomy and physiology accessible to general readers. Parker combines detailed visuals with straightforward text to explain how the body works, including both normal function and common disorders.

6. *Understanding the Human Body: An Introduction to Anatomy and Physiology* by Bruce Grice (The Teaching Company, Great Courses, 2019) Originally developed as a lecture series, this book breaks down complex physiological concepts into understandable segments using everyday examples and clear explanations. Grice takes readers through each body system, explaining how they work individually and together, while avoiding excessive medical terminology.

RECOMMENDED PODCASTS

1. "Chris Macaskill - Viva Longevity!"
https://www.youtube.com/c/plantchompers
Focus: Longevity, nutrition, factual medical science
Format: Entertaining facts, interviews with experts on aging, nutrition, metabolism and more.

2. Nicolas Verhoeven "physionic.org"
https://www.youtube.com/channel/UCj3p_1jOCJXB_L_we-DjLbA
Focus: Health optimization, medical science, physiology
Format: Deep-dive interviews with experts on metabolism, aging, nutrition, and exercise

3. "Peter Attia - The Drive"
https://peterattiamd.com/podcast/
Focus: Longevity, health optimization, medical science
Format: Deep-dive interviews with experts on metabolism, aging, nutrition, and exercise

4. "Found My Fitness with Dr. Rhonda Patrick"
https://www.foundmyfitness.com/podcast
Focus: Aging, nutrition, genetics, exercise science
Format: Scientific discussions and expert interviews about improving healthspan

5. "Huberman Lab"
https://hubermanlab.com/
Focus: Neuroscience, biology, practical health protocols
Format: Scientific explanations of body/brain function with actionable protocols

6. "The Longevity Now Podcast"
https://maxlugavere.com/podcast
Focus: Brain health, aging, nutrition
Format: Interviews with experts on cognitive health and longevity

7. "STEM-Talk"
https://www.ihmc.us/stemtalk/
Focus: Science, health, longevity research
Format: In-depth interviews with scientists and researchers

8. "The Lifespan Podcast with Dr. David Sinclair"

https://www.lifespanpodcast.com/
Focus: Aging research, longevity interventions
Format: Scientific discussions about aging and practical interventions

9. "The Proof with Simon Hill"
https://www.theproof.com/podcast
Focus: Evidence-based nutrition, longevity
Format: Expert, in-depth, long format interviews and scientific analysis of health research

10. "The Health Theory with Tom Bilyeu"
https://impacttheory.com/health-theory/
Focus: Health optimization, performance, longevity
Format: Interviews with health experts and thought leaders

11. "The Mindbodygreen Podcast"
https://www.mindbodygreen.com/podcast
Focus: Holistic health, wellness, longevity
Format: Conversations with health experts, doctors, and researchers

Note: Podcast availability and links may change over time. It's recommended to check current platforms like YouTube, Apple Podcasts, Spotify, or Google Podcasts for the most up-to-date access information. Also, while these podcasts provide valuable information, they should not be considered medical advice, and listeners should always consult healthcare professionals for personal medical decisions.

Printed in Dunstable, United Kingdom

63392386R00131